V for Veg

The Best of Philly's Vegan Food Column

Vance Lehmkuhl

Sullivan Street Press

Copyright @ 2016 by Vance Lehmkuhl

All rights reserved. No parts of this book may be reproduced in any form or by any means without the prior written consent of the publisher, except by a reviewer who may quote brief passages in a review.

The content of this book originally appeared in the "V for Veg" column of the Philadelphia Daily News, with the following exceptions: "Creator of 'Earthlings' looks at bigger picture in 'Unity'," "Yes, 'Noah' is totally vegan propaganda" and "Eating vegan saves 'The Martian'—and us?" originally appeared on the website Philly.com as "V for Vegan" blog posts; "Once Upon a Crime" and "The Decline & Fall of Human Supremacy" originally appeared in Vegetarian Voice, the magazine of the North American Vegetarian Society; and "On Earth Day, chew on these nutty facts" originally appeared as an op-ed in the Daily News, subsequently adapted as a blog entry on The Huffington Post.

Digital ISBN: 978–0–9963491–6–1
Print ISBN: 978–0–9963491–7–8

Printed in USA

Contents

Introduction 1

Counter Proposal

Kale Chips: Betcha Can't Eat Just One 9
You Don't Know Jack(fruit) 11
Keen on Quinoa 13
Veggies: Cake's Best Friend 15
Vegan Cheese Is Ready for Its Close-Up 17
The Widening Appeal and Scope of Raw Vegan 19
Egg-Free Solution: Vegan Cake Makers Are
    Going Gonzo for Garbanzos 21

Help Your Shelves

Vegan Sushi's on a Roll 27
Really Fresh Is Really Making Its Vegan Mark 30
This New "Fake Meat" Just Might Fool You 32
New Products Have the White Stuff to Compete 36
Silk's "Milkman" Ad Shows Nondairy Milks' Punch 38
High-End Almond Milk Not as Nutty an Idea as You'd Think 40
Without Fish, Plenty More Food in the Sea 43

Personalities

Cory Booker Goes Vegan: "I Wasn't Living My Truth"..........49

Foer's Crusade: Famed Author Uses His
    Pen to Challenge Meaty Status Quo 52

A Meal Where Jews, Non-Jews and Turkeys All Give Thanks......55

For Mayim Bialik, It's Vegan Parenting First,
    Neuroscience Second..............................57

Friends, Not Food 60

Stewarts as Stewards................................64

Eating Clockwise...................................68

Neal Barnard's Book Is Full of Food for Thought.............71

Creator of *Earthlings* Looks at Bigger Picture in *Unity*.........75

Five Reasons the Pope Should Eat Vegan in Philly............77

Vegan in the World

Past Presidents' Precedents for Veganism 83

Elbows without Grease 86

On a Tight Budget? Lose That Pricey Meat 91

Vegetarian + Love: Can Couples Make It Work? 93

Will New Dietary Guidelines Survive Big Meat's Ire? 95

Veganism: The "Whole" Picture 97

Pssst, Deen Foes: "Vegan" and "Healthy" Are Not Synonyms.....104

Food Faves

Vegan Thanksgiving: From Tofurky to the Three Sisters........109

Keeping the Soul, Losing the Meat......................111

Putting the "Fun" in Fungi 113
Vegan Boy Meets Grill. 117
Still Time to Rake in Your Own Fresh Veggies 119
Get Fruit and Veggies the Easy Way: Drinking 121
Rock the Crock. 124
Recipe Remakes for Vegan Junk-Food Junkies 128
No Harm, No Fowl. 130

Philly-Centric

Ready to Vedge. 137
More African-Americans Turning
  Diets Around 143
Vegan Food Traveler Finds Philly's among the Best 145
Pat's Steaks Owner: Vegan Cheesesteaks
  Even Better This Year. 147
Meatless but "Meaty" Meatballs a
  Superior Experience 149
Meatless Monday Resolution—a Good First Step, But 152
Philly Bar Scene Is Beginning to
  Embrace Veg-Head Customers 155
Vegan Pizza's So Hot, It Has a Day 157
Magic Chefs. 159
Another Philadelphia First: Birthplace of U.S. Veganism 163

The Big Picture

Yes, *Noah* Is Totally Vegan Propaganda 169
Eating Vegan Saves *The Martian*—and Us? 173

Once Upon a Crime 175
On Earth Day, Chew on These
   Nutty Facts 182
The Decline and Fall of Human Supremacy. 185

Appendix. 195

Introduction
Animal-Free News

Believe it or not, I was once a quiet, shy vegetarian.

I grew up drawing cartoon animals, and that may have been what got me interested in the minds and lives of real-life "dumb" animals. The more I learned about them, the more it seemed they were being intentionally, and unfairly, underestimated.

After years of guilt over that unfairness, I finally attempted to live my ethics in 1985, ditching meat for good. This was right after I'd moved to Philadelphia, and I spent my first five meat-free years kind of laying low, getting used to my new life.

But I guess I grew out of the quiet and shy thing: In 1990 the *Philadelphia Inquirer* played at the top of its editorial page my letter proposing "the voluntary abolition of zoos." Right at that time I also became the *Philadelphia City Paper*'s political cartoonist, a position I would hold at the alt-weekly for 12 years, drawing whatever I could get a good sociopolitical laugh out of in "How-To Harry."

I kept an eye out for issues that tied in with a pro-animal theme. The 1993 E. coli outbreak at Jack In The Box turned into "What's Really in That Burger?"—which, like so many of these cartoons, took its cue from *MAD Magazine,* furnishing "snappy answers" to the question at hand. When Florida Hispanics' ritual holiday slaughtering of goats and chickens upset mainstream America, I worked to upset them further by comparing that to the ritual holiday slaughtering of turkeys. "How-To Harry" was followed and superseded by "Edgy Veggies," my cartoon that ran in *VegNews* from 2000 to 2008.

Also in 2000, I landed my dream job as online editor at the *Philadelphia Daily News* and after a year talked them into letting me write an article about eating vegan—which I was lucky enough to see touted on the front page of the paper. Right there next to the *Daily News* logo in the corner was a banner blaring "When a Vegetarian Comes to Dinner."

Of course, back then no one would put "When a Vegan Comes to Dinner" on the front of a big-city tabloid newspaper—who would even know what you were talking about? My editors insisted on a sidebar explaining what "vegan" is and how it differs from vegetarian.

So, given the times, it was a great thing to get that visibility, spreading the word on the cover of Philly's most-read newspaper, even if the word was "vegetarian."

That was then. Now Philadelphia is a vegan-friendly mecca—our own tourism agency underscores this in pitching the city to visitors. Vedge, the city's upscale and exquisite "vegetable restaurant," continually picks up local and national honors on its way to becoming world famous. And whether they like it or not, people everywhere are becoming familiar with the word and meaning of "vegan."

I've been fortunate to keep track of progressive vegan-friendly milestones in the *Daily News,* moving from the occasional food story to vegan-issue op-eds and eventually, in July of 2011, to my column "V for Veg." This collection of vegan-Philly snapshots, nearly all from that column, tracks happenings, food trends, stories, celebrities and ideas seen through a vegan journalistic lens.

Though my driving impulse in carving out this beat was to share information and ideas, I wound up learning a hell of a lot.

I learned how to make kale chips, smoothies and jackfruit tacos; how Ben Franklin introduced tofu to the United States; how the water from a can of beans can make meringue and so many other things; how the "three sisters" tie into Thanksgiving; how people like Cory Booker, Mayim Bialik and Jonathan Safran Foer integrate their own flavors of veganism into their lives. And I learned that Philadelphia is ground zero for the vegan movement in America.

It's been great fun so far, and after nearly five years and more than a hundred columns I have at least a few dozen that I think are worth rereading, or if you're not a regular *Daily News* reader, reading for the first time.

As I said, these are snapshots, capturing vegan moments that are sometimes very specific, but I tried to pick those that have a larger point and wider appeal. I left out those columns that were too focused on one particular point in time or space, and even with those included I excised bits of now-irrelevant info, such as "upcoming" appearances by a given author.

Very occasionally I changed a word or phrase or moved a punctuation mark in attempting to make the prose as clear and useful as possible. Most of the column headlines are verbatim from their original in-paper appearance, but every once in a while I felt the brash cleverness of the *Daily News* headline-writers (e.g. "Vegans Don't Have to Cut the Cheese") was less helpful in this format than a more simple, straightforward title.

• • •

I've contributed to a half-dozen different books over the years, but this is just my second as author, and it's certainly worth mentioning my first—*The Joy of Soy*, a 1997 collection of vegetarian cartoons I'd drawn.

For that slim volume I did a series of readings around Philadelphia, in bookstores and similar venues, often featuring an improv-cartooning routine I called "Drawalong." In early 1998 my publisher, Roz Warren, alerted me to a vegetarian conference in western Pennsylvania, for which she'd chip in on registration if I went and promoted the book.

Sounded like a good idea to me, and I even talked them into letting me do a Drawalong, but soon after arriving in Johnstown, PA, I realized the awful truth: This so-called "Vegetarian Summerfest" was actually lousy with VEGANS—just the kind of people I wanted to avoid: pushy, humorless, maniacal, out of touch with day-to-day reality!

That, at least, was my understanding from years of mainstream caricatures. But spending a long weekend with these actual people—fun, friendly, pragmatic, gentle, reasonable and knowledgeable—convinced me I'd bought a load of hogwash about veganism.

I learned the now-obvious fact that cows don't simply "give" milk without giving birth; I learned the non-obvious fact that just-hatched male chicks are ground alive in what is to this day an everyday egg-industry practice. I learned that my 1985 "live my ethics" jump didn't land me where I thought it did, that where I really wanted to be was here: vegan.

But fearful of lacking the willpower to live without cheese (OMG!!!) if I went vegan overnight, I gave myself a generous 3 years to complete a gradual transition. After all, once I crossed that line I would be living the rest of my life without cheeeese!

I did gradually cut out eggs and dairy and once vegan, I was surprised after a while that I didn't need any willpower at all to avoid eating cheese—what a gross, superfluous substance it now seemed. It boggled my mind—and still does—that I had truly believed eating curdled breast milk from an animal was the height of taste-satisfaction and gustatory perfection.

So as of this writing I've been happily vegan for 15 years. But now, from my perspective as a vegan, *The Joy of Soy* is rather embarrassing.

There's a cartoon where a woman asks her waiter if the diner has a vegetarian menu and he runs and gets it and it only has one item, in huge letters: Grilled Cheese Sandwich. At the time I drew it, that seemed to really hit home—but I look at that now and I'm like, oh please, you're limited to that? Cry me a river, lady.

Another cartoon mocks a vegan hysterically concerned that cookware has been used to cook animal parts. This is what I believed vegans to be—extremists just looking for excuses to be offended. Now, of course, I'm living up to that stereotype by finding my own cartoons offensive.

So as big a part as *The Joy of Soy* played in my veganizing, it's obsolete as a calling card for my vegan take on the world. I'm hoping that although it has relatively few pictures as compared to the previous book, this one will give anyone who picks it up a good idea of both Philly's plant-based progress and my own vegan perspective.

• • •

I called this introduction "Animal-Free News." But as my insightful wife Cynthia pointed out, I'm ALWAYS going on about animals.

Guilty as charged, but as you'll notice in reading these pieces, I rarely discuss nonhuman animals themselves. I stick with human animals and the food we can eat that is free of animal parts and animal products. So in that way the phrase fits.

And the larger meaning is the point behind writing these columns in the first place. We can argue the meaning of "animal rights" till we're blue in the face (enough for a whole 'nother book), but it's abundantly clear that all of us, both human animals and nonhuman, want very much to be free to live our own lives.

So although I'm upset by food animals' captivity (not to mention the violence and cruelty visited on them on top of that), I'm grateful that I happened to be born a human and have had the freedom to write so extensively on a topic I care about, and I have to credit the *Philadelphia Daily News* as the paper that had the guts to publish it.

So I hope reading *V for Veg* (the book—and the ongoing column at Philly.com/vforveg) will bring a chuckle along with a new idea here or there. And I hope that these words and the developments they chronicle might play some part in the gradual, ongoing cultural change that eventually frees all animals.

COUNTER PROPOSAL

Kitchen Food Trends

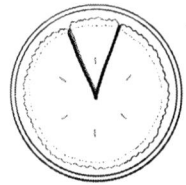

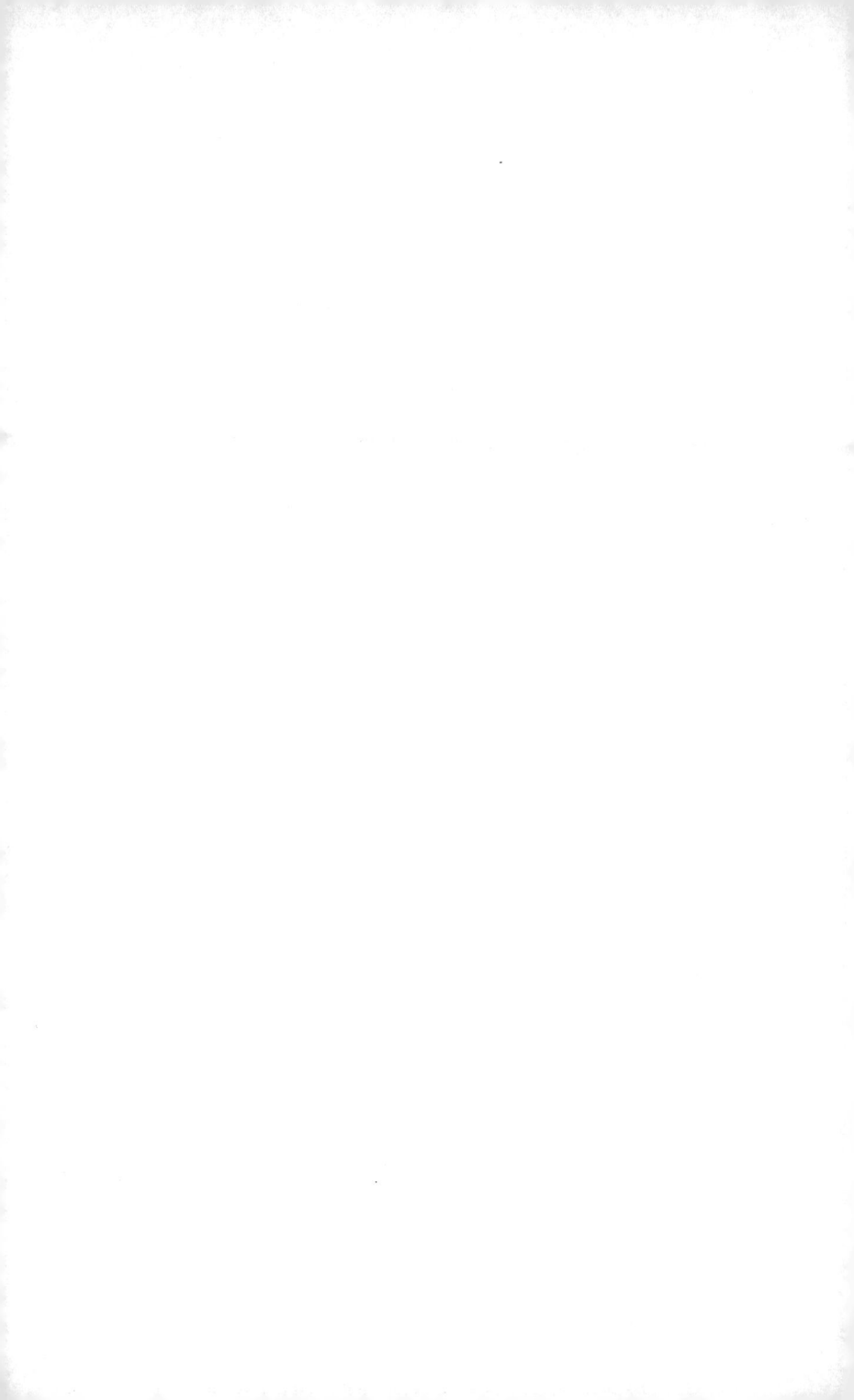

Sep 22, 2011
Kale Chips: Betcha Can't Eat Just One

Technically, kale is not a "superfood."

This cabbage-like leaf, rich in cancer-busting antioxidants and crunchy goodness, is in a class by itself, of "Super-Duper-food."

And now a super-duper-fun way to enjoy it is catching on: kale chips.

I noticed the kale-chip trend when Michele Simon, author of *Appetite for Profit* (Nation Books), tweeted about making them and got a crush of replies from people, including me, who either had also just done so or wanted to.

By the time I'd made my first batch, it seemed everybody was on the kale-chip bandwagon. Even trend arbiter Martha Stewart spotlights "kale crisps" in her 2011 "Holiday Halloween" issue of *Martha Stewart Living.*

Some stores sell premade chips for jaw-dropping prices, but you can easily make them fresh at home. It's simple: Wash a bunch of kale; dry and tear the leaves into small pieces. Put kale and some olive oil (I used a tablespoon of oil per head of kale) into a bowl and mix until the pieces are lightly coated. Season as you like (see below), then lay the pieces on a lightly greased baking tray.

The last step is heating them, and here's where methods diverge: True connoisseurs use dehydration (low heat over a long period of time), while those of us who either are impatient or don't own a dehydrator go for baking. Here, the most common formula is 425 degrees for 5–7 minutes.

Add a little salt when they come out of the oven, but not before, as it will leach moisture and make the chips more chewy than crispy. Garlic powder and dried onion added zing to mine, but try out different spicing options before baking: paprika, basil, curry or chipotle powder, sesame or cumin seeds—you name it.

Dr. Michael Greger is one of the connoisseurs. Though I called him for vitamin info (his site NutritionFacts.org features a new, entertaining video every day on the latest science in nutrition), he volunteered, "I bought a dehydrator for one purpose only, and that's to make kale chips."

He also confirmed the trend. "I did a Google image search on 'kale chips' a year ago and found almost nothing. Try it now and... wow!" (About 174,000 results, says Google.)

But my question was, are these tasty, crunchy, addictive snacks really that much healthier than, say, potato chips? The short answer? Oh, my lord, yes.

Kale chips have three times as much calcium as potato chips, four times the vitamin C, 200 times (!) the vitamin K and 400 percent (vs. 0 percent) of your daily value of vitamin A, along with other nutritive benefits. Potato chips have 20 times the calories and 100 times the fat of kale chips. So, yeah, kale makes an honest-to-goodness healthy snack chip.

I did my first couple of batches using regular curly kale, but as Martha Stewart used dinosaur (lacinato) kale, I tried that and found it much easier to render into flat strips. Either way, the baked kale has a somewhat sweet flavor that we don't usually associate with this bitter green.

One last incentive: Greger is so cuckoo for kale chips, he'll send a free DVD of his hilariously educational nutrition-fact presentations to anyone who sends him homemade kale chips. Want some nourishment news? Get cookin'!

Jun 13, 2013
You Don't Know Jack(fruit)

I've heard jackfruit called "the next kale"—a food trend ready to break wide. Which is, frankly, hard to believe.

I mean, we're talking about a huge, ungainly fruit that's sometimes 3 feet long, can weigh 80 pounds and is covered with tiny, unwelcoming spikes. When ripe, it smells like rotting onions. Cut one open and it oozes white latex that will leave you a sticky, gooey mess unless you oil your hand and your knife first. Plus, while plentiful in tropical zones, it hasn't been easy to find elsewhere.

So what's in the plus column? I'm told it has a pleasantly fruity flavor when ripe, and, hundreds of years ago, someone found that this fruit, in its unripe state, can be used in place of meat.

A versatile, chewy tabula rasa for spices, it can be used in curries but also in sloppy Joes. Known as "vegetable meat" in multiple languages, it's now showing up in blogs, cookbooks and even local menus serving just that purpose. And it has a "natural" advantage over processed meat substitutes: It's low in fat, calories and sodium, and high in vitamin C. (It is, of course, lower in protein—about 3 grams per cup.)

In the spirit of experiment, I had to try this oddity.

The first thing I learned was that there are two distinct jackfruits: One is the ripe fruit, used in sweet dishes. Canned in syrup, this is pretty widely available—I found it at all the Chinatown markets I checked—but it's not what we're looking for here.

That would be the "young green," not-quite-ripe fruit, canned in water, for which I trekked to South Philly. The two big Asian supermarkets on Washington Avenue have many different kinds of canned, unripe jackfruit, as well as whole jackfruits. I literally staggered when I saw this thing, twice as big as a prizewinning watermelon.

The raw item has a texture like artichokes but pulls into shreds instead of sheets. The flavor is mild to nonexistent, which is why most recipes start by either rubbing spices into the pieces or marinating them. Like tofu, it makes a good base for other flavors, but it also has a pleasant chewability.

I went with the most forgiving format I had heard of for jackfruit: tacos. I marinated the pieces in a barbecue-like mixture for a scant 20 minutes or so, then sautéed them with onions, breaking them into shreds with the spatula and adding a bit more barbecue sauce. I then baked the mixture for 15 minutes.

The result? Well, by the time we added fixins, these were some very good, tasty, credible tacos. Not bad for an experiment—and for a fruit subbing for meat!

But it's doubtless best tried when prepared by a pro. At Memphis Taproom, they've had Old Bay Jackfruit Cakes—the fruit subbing for crab—on the menu for about five years, according to chef Jessie Kimball.

Similarly, Mark McKinney, who oversees the menus at the Cantinas Dos Segundos and Los Caballitos, features jackfruit tacos occasionally.

I asked for prepping advice.

"We rub it with a mix of ancho and chipotle powder, cumin, paprika, black pepper and kosher salt," he explained. Then, after blackening/searing on the plancha, the fruit is braised in a basic salsa verde till it becomes tender and starts to shred like meat.

"To order, we pan-sear it in an oil infused with Mexican oregano and garlic, put it on corn tortillas and garnish with onion, cilantro and lime. Simple!"

That's the good news. The better news is that McKinney put jackfruit tacos back on the Dos Segundos and Los Caballitos menus to give "V for Veg" readers a chance to get their jackfruit feet wet.

Aug 11, 2011
Keen on Quinoa

"The Question" has been around for a while. Back in the mid-'80s, I must have been vegetarian for a good 72 hours before I first heard it.

You know the one: "Where do you get your protein?"

I guess the logical equation for meat-eaters is that, since meat is rich in protein, a diet without it must be deficient in this essential nutrient, unless there's some secret, quasi-magical source veggie folks have for procuring it. Well, folks, yes, there is indeed a secret, quasi-magical source of veggie protein, and I'm going to break the code of silence and share it with you. Ready?

It's quinoa (pronounced KEEN-wah). Used as a grain but actually the seed of a flowering plant, quinoa is packed with protein. It's a good source of iron—and it's gluten-free. It can be used in place of rice or as the main ingredient in pasta. And suddenly, it's everywhere.

Philly-area eateries such as Green Eggs Cafe, Alma de Cuba, Fork, La Copine and Pure Fare are putting their signature spin on quinoa dishes. There are also an increasing number of prepackaged quinoa products in trendy supermarkets.

But you don't need a special package to make it at home. Dynise Balcavage's *The Urban Vegan* cookbook (Three Forks) has a couple of quinoa recipes, and its author told me, "I often keep a pot of cooked quinoa in my fridge to add heft to salads and soups, or to use as a quick, nutritious side.

"Try cooking quinoa in vegetable or mushroom broth instead of water," she added. "It's a quick way to infuse it with loads of flavor."

Dynise provided a recipe for Tri-Color Quinoa, which "reminds me of a Mexican or Italian flag, with bits of kale and carrot adding texture, flavor and color."

Now that we gave quinoa its "superfood" props, here's the real secret: We don't need a special superfood.

There are tons of other solid sources of veg protein, including tofu, beans, seitan, tempeh, soy milk, peanut butter, sunflower seeds—heck, even a bagel has 9 grams of protein.

Truth is, protein is available in many foods, and Americans eat way more than we need. Pro athletes and pregnant women need more, but many of us are already consuming pregnant-athlete portions.

And forget about "combining" proteins: If you eat a variety of whole foods each day (i.e. not soda and corn chips), they'll add up to provide the whole set of amino acids that are found in meat.

Also, since it's now proven (sorry, Dr. Atkins) that weight management is all about calorie intake, it makes sense to get as much protein as you can for the smallest number of calories. And per calorie, spinach and broccoli are more of a protein powerhouse than porterhouse.

So yeah: That's where.

Feb 7, 2013

Veggies: Cake's Best Friend

I saw an ad the other day pushing bacon as an ideal Valentine's Day gift, and I had to laugh. It's like saying, "Here, sweetheart, I want you to die sooner!"

OK, I know this holiday is not about eating "right." It's about something bigger, and that something is love. Love and chocolate.

Dark chocolate is the treat that loves you back. Healthwise, you can have your chocolate cake and eat it too, especially if you mix it with—don't laugh—fruits and veggies.

It's not a new idea. In 2007, Jerry Seinfeld's wife, Jessica, smuggled "sneaky beets" into chocolate cake with her *Deceptively Delicious* cookbook (William Morrow) and recipes. Decades earlier, at least one woman, who shall remain unnamed, repeatedly and tirelessly cooked up zucchini- and spinach-laced chocolate cakes for her hapless kids, a trauma from which they're likely still reeling. (Hi, Mom!)

But there is a trend: The queen of fine vegan chocolate, Allison Rivers Samson, has noted "a recent revolution in salty and spicy chocolate flavors." She's added chipotle cinnamon fudge to her Allison's Gourmet line. In this fudge, "warming cinnamon adds extra depth while a touch of chipotle chili spices it up without setting your mouth ablaze."

In addition to side-by-side counterpoint, chocolate can blend with other flavors like, say, avocado.

Seriously.

"Avocado has a subtle taste that's easily overpowered by the strong flavor of chocolate" said Carley Leibowitz, a baker and sous chef for Miss Rachel's Pantry in South Philly. Her specialty is chocolate-avocado brownies. "Having the avocado in there adds moisture and helps the brownie to hold together better and not get crumbly."

Leibowitz adds that with avocado in the mix, "you're replacing some of the unhealthy saturated fats [plentiful in eggs and butter] with healthy, monounsaturated fats. Plus you're getting vitamin C, minerals and fiber."

OK, sure, a "healthful" brownie is better than the "death wish" valentine mentioned above, but what about chocolaty flavor? I had to try one of Leibowitz's creations.

Wow! It was gone before I could even remember to try to taste the avocado. Just as Leibowitz promised, the final product was "creamy, moist and delicious."

Fudge and brownies, mainstays of V-Day home baking, come together in black-bean brownies. In *The Happy Herbivore* (Ben-Bella), Lindsay S. Nixon adapted this counterintuitive combo into a healthful and tasty treat: Hers are animal-free, gluten-free, low-fat and high-protein, all while delivering real chocolate brownie flavor.

Nixon says she had her own sweetheart sample the batter and the finished product before she disclosed "the magical ingredient," and he "had no clue!"

There are plenty of other offbeat ways you can make chocolate say "I love you, and I want you to live forever." Chocolate, after all, has numerous proven health benefits—as long as it's vegan. Dairy seems to block or negate almost all the positive effects.

Fortunately, dark, vegan varieties are becoming more common. With such a diverse array of wacky options to mix with dark chocolate—we didn't even get to carrots, pumpkin or sweet potatoes—why choose products created from some animal's breast milk?

Feb 21, 2013

Vegan Cheese Is Ready for Its Close-Up

"Oh my God, I couldn't live without cheese!"

Ever heard those words—or maybe uttered them yourself?

I sure have. Back when I, a longtime vegetarian, decided to go vegan, the prospect of life without cheese yawned as a desolate, ascetic slog of eternity without such rich, gooey gustatory pleasure. What a martyr to cross the line into that bleak, barren world!

A couple of dairy-free months later, I was already puzzling at such grandiosity. Cheese? Really? I didn't know then how casomorphins, a dairy component that's concentrated in cheese, can act as opioids—that is, they confer a mild but habit-forming euphoria.

I wound up expanding my palate to other food combinations, never missing cheese, never trying to replace it or replicate its dishes. Good thing, too, because in those days vegan cheese was more of an earnest science-fair project than an object of desire.

Now, though, Daiya, Tofutti, Follow Your Heart and other brands have brought credible vegan cheese to the marketplace and helped drive it forward. Formerly packing animal-based casein, Galaxy Foods now has a whole line of vegan shredded cheeses you can get at the Acme.

The Acme!

The even-better news is that you can make animal-free cheese at home with help from an increasing number of food writers. I have had great results with local blogger Lee Khatchadourian's simple almond feta recipe, which you can find at Philly.com/almondfeta.

The DIY trail was blazed in 1994 by Jo Stepaniak's *Uncheese Cookbook* (Book Publishing Co.), which focused mainly on sauces, spreads and gooey soft cheeses, acquainting many with the "cheezy" properties of nutritional yeast.

Two decades later, Stepaniak is the editor on a new work, also from Book Publishing Co., that raises the bar of vegan cheese—Miyoko Schinner's *Artisan Vegan Cheese*. Here you'll find hard, sliceworthy cheeses like sharp cheddar, Parmesan and hard gruyere that achieves its cheesiness through aging over several days. There are also softer, often quicker options like tofu ricotta, meltable muenster, Camembert and cream cheese. (See her recipe for Philadelphia-style cream cheese at Philly.com/miyoko.)

Schinner's no novice when it comes to vegan cookbooks: She wrote her first one 23 years ago. But she waited to do cheese so she'd have time to experiment. She spent a year testing, tweaking, aging and air-drying many substances to arrive at nondairy cheeses that rival their animal-milk counterparts.

Her confections often use cashews, which are "a neutral-flavor nut that's soft and relatively high in fat," and "cultured, nondairy yogurt because it's already cultured, giving a head start on the whole aging process."

Sometimes, though, you don't want neutral.

"The provolone uses pine nuts because their nuttiness really adds to the flavor." And nuts are ill-suited for meltable cheeses, she pointed out, because their fat is "a solid substance that cannot get any softer."

Thanks to Schinner's expert approach, *Artisan Vegan Cheese* has both vegans and mainstream foodies raving. She reflected that "most people say, 'I could give up meat, but I couldn't live without cheese.'"

Sounds vaguely familiar.

If you're someone who's uncomfortable with the cruelty behind the production of cheese, but feel you can't live without it . . . well, you may not have to!

Apr 3, 2014
The Widening Appeal and Scope of Raw Vegan

Now that spring is finally taking hold, our fancies naturally turn from warming comfort foods to the colorful allure of fresh fruits and vegetables. Good thing, especially for those of us whose comfort was converted into a few extra pounds over the winter.

It's a good time to check out some of the freshest, most colorful cuisine, which is raw.

OK, I hear ya. After all, "raw" to us vegans is like "vegan" is to the rest of the world: An imponderable extreme that we know is probably better in many ways, but who can live like that? I mean, what is there left to eat?

Lisa Ransing, of Full Moon Fare, is ready with answers, in the form of zucchini noodles with creamy cashew alfredo sauce, BBQ kale chips, fruit salad with coconut almond crisps, walnut/hempseed/mushroom burgers with eggplant "bacon," goji superfood bars, tacos with "nacho cheese" sauce, super salad with sprouted quinoa and pumpkin seeds, and lemon lavender cream tarts—to name a few of the items on this week's menu.

Of course, variety is pointless unless it tastes great, and having tried Full Moon's fare, I can assure you it delivers in more ways than one. Twice a week, within Philadelphia, FMF brings a box with four entrees, two breakfast items, kale chips and a dessert for $100. I found the sample box from a recent weekly menu so varied, creative and delicious I had to keep reminding myself I was eating "raw food."

Considering Ransing's kitchen pedigree, this is no surprise: In a phone interview she mentioned an eight-year stint with Georges Perrier, working "in all his restaurants" at one time or another, where she learned "all the different possible flavors" that she now combines in fascinating ways.

As "more of a chef than a nutritionist," Ransing leaves the discussion of enzyme depletion and fiber abundance to others, focusing on getting raw foods into people's mouths, where it sells itself.

"I love introducing people to whole food," she said, "and desserts is a good place to start. Whenever I'm giving somebody something for the first time, I give them desserts."

We're not talking fruit cups, but fully realized concoctions such as cheesecake and avocado-infused key lime pie. Ransing gets a special kick, she said, "when people say, 'I don't like raw food,' and they try it, and like it."

That seems to be happening more and more. Whether for health reasons or simple, fresh tastiness, raw food is gaining ground. Ransing observes that "just over the past two years, the amount of raw food available in town has really increased. I think Philadelphia's ready for an all-raw restaurant."

While Ransing and her partner, Michael Waring, pursue that goal, they're concentrating on delivery, catering and events like the yoga dinner "Namaste for Dinner." Yoga teacher Gabrielle Sigal leads an hour-and-45-minute class, followed by an all-vegan buffet—and "people get to take home the leftovers," Ransing noted.

In that case, you may want to "spring" onto this opportunity, because if I show up, there may not be any leftovers.

Dec 4, 2015
Egg-Free Solution: Vegan Cake Makers Are Going Gonzo for Garbanzos

Planning holiday baking? Then you're probably all too aware that many people (family members?) are ditching eggs for various reasons.

For some it's allergies, for some the massive cholesterol, for others the massive cruelty, for still others the government/industry dirty tricks to squelch egg-free competition.

And let's not forget the increased costs from bird flu, or the fact that a surprising number of folks just don't like the taste of eggs.

Yet, eggless baking options have been less than perfect, with different substitutions for different functions. If only there were one solution that was animal-free, gluten-free, cholesterol-free, worry-free and, well . . . free!

There is: It's the slimy water in a can of chickpeas.

You read right: The "food waste" that you're about to pour down the drain when you use the garbanzos (or any other kind of bean) is aquafaba. It's taking the eggless baking world by storm, and whatever you're planning to bake, it can help you pull it off with zero eggs.

Outside of a couple of isolated one-shots, this "new" food technology is just one year old. French tenor and gourmet Joël Roessel came up with the idea of whipping chickpea "jus" as a foundation (along with other ingredients) for chocolate mousse and similar desserts, and published his results in December 2014 on his site,

Revolution Vegetale. A couple of months later, two French vegan hipsters presented an eerily similar process on their YouTube show, and a Seattle software engineer named Goose Wohlt saw it.

Wohlt had already been experimenting to create a vegan meringue and was intrigued by the chickpea-juice concept. As a true methodical engineer, "I started with only granulated sugar & well-strained chickpea liquid to see how just those two ingredients would interact," he told me via email, "and it just worked." After all these years and tears, all you needed was chickpea juice, sugar and some serious whipping action.

Wohlt posted his discovery on Facebook, where Rebecca August, an animal-care worker from Michigan, saw it and suggested that they launch "another [Facebook] group dedicated to this miracle liquid," she told me, adding that "Goose was very intent on making it an open-sharing development group, so that is the way it was set up from the beginning." A veteran forum admin, August has kept the "Vegan Meringue—Hits and Misses" discussion focused on vegan foods, spurning larger animal-free philosophy discussions.

As the group got going, Wohlt coined the term "aquafaba" for the chickpea juice and its associated culinary realm. Over the course of the year, amateur chefs and bakers joined and shared both success stories and, well, misses, when the results didn't pan out, with the group pitching in to try to figure out which tweaks would make it work the next time. As of this writing, the group has 31,000 members.

Meanwhile, it turns out that aquafaba does way more than meringues. August said that after mastering them, "I went pretty quickly into baking cakes with it," finding, as many have, that it helps baked goods rise and hold together while remaining light, moist and fluffy. August added that "after about the first two months of experimenting, I think I'd eaten about 10 pounds of sugar, and backed off pretty strongly after that."

Fortunately, the Facebook community took over the heavy lifting and by now there are well over 100 recipes collected on the group's page—not just for mousse and lemon-meringue pies but muffins, doughnuts, brownies, Yorkshire pudding, challah, nougat, cookies (dozens of varieties), cakes (from mud to sponge to carrot), custard, mayonnaise, quiche and even butter and cheese. The list of "aquafabized" foods keeps growing, with the holy grail of angel-food cake finally looking like it may be conquered this month.

The fun isn't limited to baking: One high-profile group member, Vegan Street's Marla Rose, used an aquafaba wash to add a lustrous golden brown finish to her phyllo-based Thanksgiving centerpiece (soft-pretzel vendors, take note!). Other innovations and improvements continue to show up daily.

In Philadelphia the word is just getting around, with some vegan bakers reporting initial efforts and others saying "aqua-whuzzah?"

Vegan doyenne Christina Pirello has achieved "spectacular results" in a cake: "I used 1/3-cup for every egg. No odd flavor, and the cake really rose." Since she uses coconut sugar, though, she said her meringue came out runny. Meanwhile, over at Naturally Sweet Desserts, Sherimane Johnson likes it for whipped cream: "After 15 minutes of whipping garbanzo bean brine with cream of tartar and sugar you get a gorgeous, shiny, marshmallow-fluff-type product." She warns that if it sits out too long "it begins to return to liquid."

I know one vegan baker who made two batches of peanut-butter cookies a week apart, the second with aquafaba, and said the latter cookies held together distinctly better than those made with traditional starch-based egg replacer. My wife, Cynthia, made some delicious, moist gingerbread using an old recipe with the standard substitution of 3 tablespoons to replace one egg. I made some tasty oil-free chocolate-chip cookies (from Goose Wohlt's recipe) that use both the aquafaba and the chickpeas themselves—and it occurred to me that the delicious cookies I just tried from Hungryroot, a vegan-friendly delivery service, also were made with chickpeas, so who knows how far this trend is spreading?

Wohlt's site, aquafaba.com, has a donate button for the lab tests that will nail down the chemical constituency of aquafaba (at a "nutrition facts" level) and further research will pinpoint exactly what is going on chemically with this "magic" ingredient. A cookbook may also be in the works, but Wohlt says his priority is to update aquafaba.com with a recipe-search tool and individual recipe commenting to spread the word beyond Facebook, and also because "the FB 'Files and Posts' interface is severely limited."

The takeaway from all this is that another longtime pillar of animal-based food, with all its associated liabilities, turns out to be totally unnecessary, easily replaced in rarefied confections by a whole-food plant product that you were going to throw away. And that's great news for anyone who wants to make treats everyone can enjoy, while truly celebrating peace on earth.

HELP YOUR SHELVES

The Vegan Marketplace

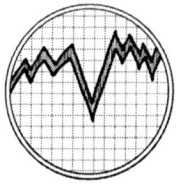

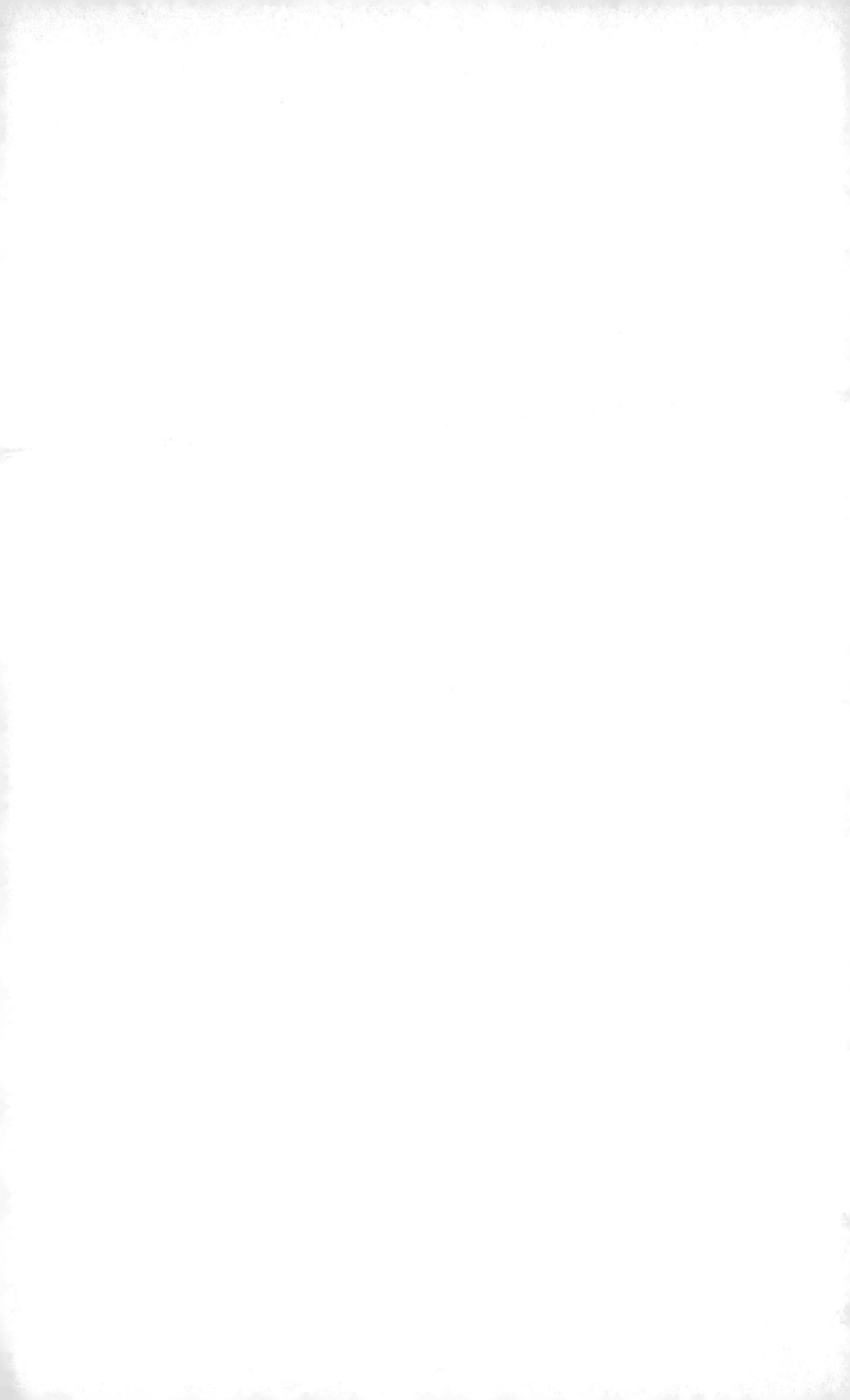

Jul 27, 2012
Vegan Sushi's on a Roll

Say the words "vegan sushi" to your average fine-diner and you're likely to get a blank stare. How, after all, can anything be called sushi without raw fish, the very meaning of the word itself?

Actually, the word sushi does not refer to raw fish, but to the key ingredient, vinegared rice. That's what makes sushi sushi.

This comes up now for two reasons: One is that these hot July days are a perfect time to enjoy the cool pleasures of this Japanese staple; the other is that the fish-free-sushi envelope is being pushed in a big way by the appropriately named Beyond Sushi, which opened this month in New York City and is drawing crowds.

"I think it's a very mainstream thing," said Guy Vaknin, the "Hell's Kitchen" star behind the restaurant. He does admit that "some people tell me it's not really sushi at all. I say, that's fine, that's why I call it Beyond Sushi."

Vaknin is one pioneer within a wave of veg-friendly sushi styles that have grown in popularity within the past few years, a microcosm of sushi's burgeoning popularity worldwide over the past quarter-century or so.

But these veggie elements were always there within the sushi tradition: For instance, there's a style of sushi roll called futomaki whose most common varieties are vegetarian, combining multiple innards like cucumber, bamboo shoots, pickled daikon and diced carrots. Other varieties may include cooked crab, fish paste or pieces of omelet.

As more people in the U.S. are replacing animal products with plant foods, it's worth remarking that this very process has played an important role in the development of the cuisine: The California roll, invented at the restaurant Tokyo Kaikan in the late '60s, is widely credited with expanding the appeal of sushi from Southern California—where Japanese immigrants had established a beachhead—across the rest of America and then the rest of the world.

And what was the signature innovation of the California roll? Replacing fatty tuna with avocado.

Regional variations soon spread across the U.S. One was the Philly roll, which added the namesake cream cheese. But vegan variations also emerged in places where fresh fruit and avocados are plentiful, like Hawaii.

One fun thing about sushi is that anything that can be chopped or arranged into a cylindrical pattern can be a potential filling. And almost every sushi roll has some plant element, from the more basic (asparagus, cucumber, carrots, scallions, mushrooms, tofu and bamboo shoots) to more adventurous (mango, pineapple, sweet potato, daikon and pickled plum, or umeboshi).

The veg-friendly aspect of sushi often gets overlooked, but there are plenty of reasons people may want to go fish-free. The Beyond Sushi site notes that veggie sushi is "perfect for pregnant women who cannot eat fish for 9 months and are bored with ordering mundane cucumber-avocado rolls with standard white rice," and also that "kids who don't like fish in their sushi can get their servings of fruits and veggies in a tasty way."

Of course, in addition to wanting to avoid the mercury in most fatty wild fish and the diseases of farmed fish, some choose not to eat seafood because our oceans have been overfished, or because they don't want to deprive an animal of life. Then there are simply those who say, "Raw fish? Yecch!"

So if you want veggie sushi, where do you go? Beyond Sushi is an obvious destination for the adventurous Philadelphia-area connoisseur. As part of his "beyond" approach, Vaknin uses black rice or a rice blend, and avoids soy sauce and other high-sodium elements. He depends on the freshness of ingredients and his combination of them to deliver "a burst of flavor."

It's this skill in pairing and balancing filling components that makes for a mouth-pleasing sushi experience. A vegetarian himself, Vaknin knows that "people often think something's not going to be as flavorful being vegetarian." But he's proving them wrong: "I say it's all about how much love you put into it."

Then again, not all of us are going to make the hike to Manhattan just for a roll or a hunk of nigiri (sushi comes in many formats; we're focusing on "maki" rolls). Fortunately, it's quite feasible to get interesting veg rolls at most regular sushi restaurants around Philadelphia. The one caveat is that if you're totally fish-free, you may need to ask about fish flakes in broth (dashi) or sauces that are often used to flavor the sushi ingredients.

Like soup, sushi is a forgiving food medium. Thus, anyone with a hankering for the funky finger food can make sushi at home. Although it may take a master's skill to create the colorful, eye-popping aesthetics of Beyond Sushi ("first you eat with your eyes," reminds Vaknin), you can begin with established pairings before you get adventurous.

If you know how to cook rice, you're already most of the way there. You can start with a basic, fail-safe filling combo like carrots, scallion and cucumber—balancing sweet, spicy and "clean" flavors, respectively—and then start swapping in other elements with similar properties.

The basic flavor is meant to be supplemented with a more powerful sauce, often flavored with pickled ginger or wasabi. (That's green Japanese horseradish, though any "wasabi" you're likely to get around here is really just horseradish, mustard and green coloring.)

You can also add wasabi or pickled ginger to the interior of the roll. Go ahead and dip the thing in soy sauce for one more layer of kick.

Once you have your basic ingredients—prepared rice, fillings and nori (seaweed) wrappers—the only other thing you may want to get is a small bamboo mat to help with rolling the sushi cylinder. Find them at dollar stores or supermarkets. You don't have to get an elaborate sushi-making kit for what is essentially a place mat. And if you don't have a mat, you can use a dish towel.

Whether you're trekking up to Beyond Sushi, finding veg options around town or making your sushi at home, here's one thing you don't need: chopsticks. Sushi rolls are meant to be eaten with your fingers—and with delight! So go ahead and have it your way.

Feb 6, 2014
Really Fresh Is Really Making Its Vegan Mark

"Tasty enough to turn Jay Z vegan!" That's a slogan Mickey Davis and Dorinda Hampton have not yet used to promote their Philly-based food line Really Fresh Vegan. But it's not out of the question.

Davis, a.k.a. "Black Key," is a Grammy-nominated music producer who's worked with Ludacris, 50 Cent and DMX. He told me how, as producer of the official B-side remix of Beyoncé's 2006 "Deja Vu" single (Columbia), he'd discussed vegan food with Jay Z, and got him to try some.

Whether the superstars' December "22-day vegan challenge" was inspired by Davis and Hampton may never be known—until

I get the chance to ask Jay Z himself—but Really Fresh Vegan aims for a big impact here in the Delaware Valley, where RFV sandwiches, snacks, juices and dessert items are increasingly showing up on store shelves.

"We want to reach anybody who likes food," Davis said, "not just people who think of it as vegan food."

Hampton, who perfects the recipes, agreed. "Lots of people think something weird's going on with vegan," said Hampton, a veteran of Food Network's "24-Hour Restaurant Battle." "They can't see themselves eating anything that doesn't have some kind of meat protein in it." So, she works to make animal-free offerings that compete fully alongside mainstream products.

"I make everything the star," she explained, cooking ingredients separately and "combining them slowly to build up flavor components." She knows the attention to detail has paid off when she hears, "This food tastes good," not "This vegan food tastes good."

When Hampton says that tasters "couldn't believe it had no animal products," that echoes the surprised accolades of judges in her Food Network appearance. And having enjoyed some of RFV's cookies, pies and flavored popcorn myself, I can sympathize.

The business dates back to 2011, and for much of the interim was incarnated as Sprout, a juice bar in Kennett Square. Last summer, though, they decided to close that storefront "to focus on manufacturing, to be able to reach more people," Davis said.

To that end, new products are in development, including a "hybrid" (juice + herbs + probiotics) juice cleanse called "Day" that will be delivered locally, plus a line of breakfast convenience foods targeted to busy Penn students.

On the latter, Davis credited the Penn Vegan Society with invaluable advice. For his part, Victor Galli, of PVS, recalled, "We walked into one of the retailers and saw Really Fresh Vegan, tried some of it and were impressed by how high-quality the items were."

Quality is important, Galli stressed, because eaters of vegan food "need to prove to the world that we're discerning," not just buying whatever says "vegan" on the label. (It's the same "raise the bar" impulse that drives the PVS-initiated Ivy League Vegan Conference.)

To Hampton, success is measured by the fact that "people say, 'This is a food I can eat,'" not worrying about what niche it might be filling. And the more people try and enjoy RFV, the less weird, and more mainstream, animal-free eating becomes.

As we go to press, the online buzz mill has Beyoncé starting another 22-day vegan stint after slimming down with the last one. Davis said that he wouldn't be surprised to see B remain vegan, because, with the right foods, plant-based eating sells itself.

"Even if you don't do it the whole way," he said, "you can still see benefits."

Nov 1, 2012
This New "Fake Meat" Just Might Fool You

A couple of weeks ago, I stood beside chef David Silver as he handed out samples of a new product at Whole Foods Market.

"What is it?" one gray-haired fellow inquired, taking a bite.

"It's Beyond Meat," said Silver, seeming to allow the guy another chew or two before adding, "It's a vegan meat."

Rather than responding with a comical spit-take, the man nodded cheerily and said, "Well, I don't like 'vegan'—but I like this!"

Silver has heard that a lot, traveling around the region training staff and whipping up recipes to showcase the new product, one that aspires to compete with meat on its own terms. He's aware that meat-eaters can have a knee-jerk aversion to the v-word. He's also aware that context—his flavorful sauces replicating those of favorite meat dishes—plays a big role in food tasting. And he believes this is no ordinary meat substitute.

Beyond Meat has been called "the game changer" in vegan and vegetarian diets. It has fooled some—including *New York Times* columnist Mark Bittman—into thinking they were eating actual meat. It's high in protein, low in fat, and gluten- and cholesterol-free.

And it's launching in greater Philadelphia today, which happens to be World Vegan Day. In Whole Foods stores throughout our area (and a few natural-foods stores here and there), you can now get Beyond Meat in the prepared foods section. By next weekend, this will be the case across the mid-Atlantic region.

So what is it exactly? Mostly soy protein, pea protein and carrot fiber. But what gives Beyond Meat its edge is the careful way the components are mixed, heated, cooled and shaped in a form that has much of the flavor and texture of meat—a process licensed from the University of Missouri by Ethan Brown.

"People always say, 'Why are you imitating meat?'" Brown remarked by phone. "'I thought you'd want nothing to do with meat.' But I say, why throw out all those hundreds of years of culinary development? The key is to take the animal protein out and provide the same nutritional benefits without the downsides."

Brown grew up on a farm in Maryland and spent a couple of his teenage years in the Philly suburbs. "I was a Bucks County all-star in basketball," he said. A decade ago he went vegan and began looking for a way to develop "clean, eco-friendly, high-value nutrition that takes animal welfare into account."

He's also taking the realities of the marketplace into account.

"We have a two-pronged strategy," he said of the company that makes Beyond Meat—Savage River Inc., based in El Segundo, Calif. "One, to perfectly replicate the taste and experience of eating meat, and two, to drive the retail price lower than that of meat."

Compared with raising and killing a chicken, the numbers are favorable: "It basically takes us two hours to do what takes our competition six weeks."

Now, "fake meats" are already available in stores, and they've been around for centuries, but this one has attracted a huge amount of buzz. Dan Murphy, a pro-beef columnist for cattlenetwork.com, warned his colleagues that it's "so good that even industry insiders could be fooled in a blind taste test."

Twitter co-founder Biz Stone, a vegan himself, was impressed enough to invest in the company and join the board.

Stone's Obvious Corp. seeks out new systems to make the world better, and he found that while a new kind of food was not an, um, obvious candidate at first, it wound up being a perfect fit.

"What attracted me," he told me earlier this week, "was the combination of ambition and science they had for this. It's fundamentally more than [creating] a novelty food. They want to compete directly with the meat industry."

By putting "meat" in the name, the company is throwing down the gauntlet, challenging consumers to throw out preconceptions about plant-based eating, and Stone talks about it the way some do about veganism itself.

"The goal is not to give anything up," he said. "It's to gain something. You're getting more nutrition, better health, and you're gaining efficiency."

Livestock production, of course, is a famously wasteful and inefficient way to process water and plant protein into edible food. When you look at what you're getting instead of what you're avoiding, he said, "that's a big perspective change."

Stone is confident that cruelty-free, healthy foods will continue to be a trending topic. "The general populace can do their own research, and as consumers become more aware of what's going on, that's going to make them trend toward the most humane choices," he said.

It's no secret that the case for animal-free food is getting stronger, and not just for the obvious environmental and disease-fighting benefits. This summer, leading scientists from around the world signed a "Declaration of Consciousness" for nonhuman animals, recognizing that humans' capacity for consciousness is not unique and urging the public to recognize animals' sentience. The scientist who organized the signing has since gone vegan.

Stone is looking down the road. In the long term, he said, "it's not going to work for the world to keep eating animals. There needs to be some kind of advancement."

Ethan Brown, similarly, compares the move toward plant-based "meat" to the change "from the horse-drawn carriage to the automobile." That change didn't happen overnight. But looking back now, it seems, well, obvious.

Even a half-century ago, our culture didn't grasp nutrition, environmental impacts or animal sentience the way we do now.

Who knows? Over the course of history humans have advanced beyond a lot of unsavory attitudes.

Maybe now is the time to get beyond meat.

Jan 23, 2014

New Products Have the White Stuff to Compete

So: January 23—too soon to call 2014 "the year of the vegan"? Not if you're *New York* magazine, which noted last week that "news outlets on both sides of the Atlantic" have already declared it.

And who am I to argue?

Veganism is seeping into everyday life through so many channels, it's hard to keep track of the milestones.

Two buzzed-about veganizations recently seen on Delaware Valley grocery shelves range from a jar of plain mayo to a line of artisan soft gourmet cheeses.

The more cultured of these, obviously, is the cheese. Kite Hill brought together celeb vegan chef Tal Ronnen (he helped Oprah Winfrey do a 21-day vegan cleanse and catered Ellen DeGeneres and Portia De Rossi's wedding), some other foodies and a biochemist to perfect a nutmilk-culture-enzyme combo that achieves a persuasive gourmet cheese flavor and texture. So far, three varieties are available, exclusively at Whole Foods: Casuccio, "a soft fresh with a supple, silky texture"; Costanoa, "a semi soft dusted with a piquant blend of paprika and fennel pollen"; and White Alder, "a soft ripened cheese with a delicate white rind, pungent aroma and velvety texture," according to a company press release.

I have sampled Kite Hill products, although as someone whose expert knowledge of gourmet cheese consists mostly of being able to recite Monty Python's "Cheese Sketch," I can offer only my uncultured reactions.

The White Alder and the Costanoa, tried on crackers, were pleasant enough, both rich and subtle, but they didn't exactly turn my world upside down.

The third, however, exactly did. I had one bite of the Truffle-Dill-Chive Casuccio and I immediately needed another. The dill was predominant, but the flavor quickly blossomed into delicious multiplicity.

"This is what folks like that hoity-toity John Cleese character were enthused about!" I thought.

Other types of characters—like, say, Joe Lunchbucket—might be interested in a new mayonnaise called Just Mayo that's grabbing attention from no less than Bill Gates, an investor in parent company Hampton Creek.

I tried Just Mayo in a couple of sauces, where it performed admirably, and in a sandwich (peppered Tofurky slices with shredded kale) that turned out totally delicious.

Vegan mayonnaise dates clear back to the 20th century, but the twist here is that the company first created a plant-based "egg" from which the mayonnaise is made, giving it a creamy, smooth texture and pitch-perfect taste that has won over egg-mayo adherents. The base product, Beyond Eggs, is the foundation of more offerings.

One is a cookie dough called "Eat the Dough," whose name slaps the egg industry where it hurts; eating raw egg-based dough is risky due to the prevalence of fecal bacteria. Hampton Creek aims to compete with eggs on an institutional scale and is taking no prisoners. Some Whole Foods stores are already using Just Mayo for regular deli sandwiches.

Gourmet cheese and mayo occupy nearly opposite food niches, but these new vegan versions share more than their off-white (perhaps even ecru) color: While cholesterol-free and relatively low in saturated fat and sodium, they're still full of flavor, adding zest and zing to the notion that this really may be the Year of the Vegan!

Jun 14, 2012
Silk's "Milkman" Ad Shows Nondairy Milks' Punch

If you drink cow's milk, it's likely that at one point or another you had to be talked into it. "Getting kids to drink milk" is a well-recognized meme (try Googling the phrase) in song, story and parenting guides, because the beverage is not, apparently, something we take to automatically.

But given enough "wholesome" spin (the National Dairy Council made health claims that the FTC in 2007 determined to be unfounded, forcing their retraction) and government-funded campaigns (remember the U.S. Department of Agriculture's team-up with Domino's to sell more cheese per pizza?) cow's milk has been positioned as the natural, normal drink for everybody, with soy milk as the weird upstart challenger.

That's quickly changing, though, with more varieties of plant-based milk showing up on supermarket shelves. And a new Silk ad raises the stakes by reframing dairy as the "weird" choice.

John Brookbank's 50-second spot was a finalist in last year's user-submitted contest, and though it's not scheduled for TV, it is on Silk's official YouTube channel (see it at Philly.com/almondmilk).

Riffing on a familiar theme (suddenly-appearing superhero persuades consumer to switch to new/better product), Brookbank has his "Power Milkman" knocking the milk jug from a poor schlub's hands. When the bike-messenger-outfitted superhero is told "you sure don't look like a milkman," he quips "and you sure don't look like a baby cow!"

The ad's over-the-top hilarity mixes "extreme" sound effects, cheeky puns, a fake-mustache gag and a brazen tagline, calling Silk PureAlmond "a superior product that's made for people—not suckling cows."

Whether or not that's a factor, the trends are clear: Plant-milk sales are on the rise in the U.S. while dairy continues to decline.

And the pro-dairy outfits that worked so hard to hype the supposed "dangers of soy" now must chase consumers away from almonds, rice, coconut, flax, hemp, oats, hazelnuts and others.

Almond milk is the success story of the moment; it's now available in supermarkets everywhere and challenging soy for the top spot. Coconut milk (a beverage distinct from the cooking liquid) has also made great strides in market share.

So if you're curious, which one should you try? One advantage to the multiplicity of different milks is that they excel in different situations. While I never took to soy milk on cereal—too cloying—rice milk and almond milk work wonderfully. For cooking or baking, you'll almost always want an unsweetened variety. Soy, almond and coconut all perform well. Flax milk is great in smoothies, boosting omega-3s without altering flavor (and without leaving flax seeds to clean out of your blender).

And for drinking? That will depend on your taste, as well as what you're drinking it with. I find almond and coconut both go well with cookies, while rice and oat may be better standalones, but that's subjective. I also enjoy blending the different types to get the best balance for a given occasion.

Cholesterol-free milks made from nuts, grains and legumes have been around for centuries, and the modern versions are calcium-fortified. "Superior" products? That depends, but they are made for humans, by humans.

Weird, huh?

Aug 6, 2015
High-End Almond Milk Not as Nutty an Idea as You'd Think

Thanks to hipster vegans, almond milk is suddenly a thing—and not just a thing, but a bad thing: Almonds, a "thirsty crop," are draining California's water and increasing the drought, all for a product that's only 2 percent nuts. Right?

Hang on: Actually, almond milk was "a thing" back in the middle ages, used widely because it didn't spoil as quickly as cow's milk, and because for many, almonds were easier to get than cows. And the $900 million spent on almond milk last year, making it the declining dairy industry's top competitor, came from a much larger crowd than the pool of vegans and/or hipsters.

As for water use, California's thirstiest crop by an order of magnitude is not almonds but livestock. A glass of cow's milk is more water-intensive than one of almond milk.

And as for the charge that some brands contain only 2 percent almonds, well... on that one, local almond lover Jeff Fonseca isn't arguing.

"The product they're 'destroying California' with is of such low value—the current almond milk industry is an illusion of health," he scoffed, as we sat in a Fishtown cafe.

So, Fonseca and his MBA-toting biz partner, Ryan Fitzpatrick, put their heads together to start Almond Bros., a line of almond milks made from heaping helpings of raw, organic almonds. He pegs the Bros. variety at close to 25 percent almonds. But it's more than that: "We use a specific unique almond that we get direct from a small family farm in California," he explained. "They're refrigerated right after harvesting, never treated" with chemicals or steam.

"And soaking the almonds, as we do, makes for better digestibility," he added. "It makes the skins less inhibitive of the [beneficial] enzymes in the nuts."

Fitzpatrick handed me a Mason jar of Almond Bros., and I took a swig. The concoction was lighter and simpler than the big-box almond milks I've had, not overly sweet, but flavorful. I remarked on the welcome absence of a gummy note in the texture.

"Yeah, sunflower lecithin is the only emulsifier we use," Fonseca noted. "And of course no carrageenan," said Fitzpatrick, referring to the thickener commonly used in mainstream nondairy milk and now widely seen as a health liability.

The Bros.' next step is pasteurization. They'll use a high-pressure process to maintain as much of the raw nuts' nutrition and quality as possible, Fonseca said. At that point, Almond Bros. can be sold on a per-unit basis in a retail setting, but both Bros. agree they'll move slowly and methodically to keep quality as high as possible.

For now, the main outlet is Miss Rachel's Pantry, which will offer Almond Bros. by the glass starting next week. Already Rachel Klein's multi-course farmhouse-table dinners have been featuring the product as a dessert-course accompaniment. "Being aligned with a vegan community that's so close and supportive is something that motivated us," said Fitzpatrick.

If you can't get to South Philly, or are just the DIY type, consider making your own almond milk at home with the help of Alan Roettinger's *The Almond Milk Cookbook* (Book Publishing Co.).

The guide from the prolific Mexico-raised chef and *Extraordinary Vegan* author (Book Publishing Co.) starts with the basic process of almond milk making, then moves to almond cream, and from there into salad dressings, soups, sauces, smoothies and desserts. Roettinger quips that "as my wife pointed out to me, the chocolate-almond ice cream in the book is one of the ten best things I've ever made," which might sound boastful, but I tried that ice cream at this year's Vegetarian Summerfest, and it was outstanding.

Roettinger is similarly blunt in looking at the big picture: "Almond milk is popular for a reason," he told me via email. "People are starting to realize that consuming dairy milk does NOT do a body good, and they're eager to try alternatives."

One thing sales figures make clear is that the nondairy appeal goes way beyond vegans. I first decided almond milk had cracked the mainstream when my local Super Fresh started carrying Califia almond-milk coffee creamer.

This is not to say that almond is permanently installed at the top of the heap. Coconut-based milks, creamers and especially ice creams are showing up all over.

Also coming up strong in 2015 is cashew milk, which Silk began pushing onto market shelves at the end of the last year.

Waiting in the wings are peanut milk, quinoa milk, oat, flax, hemp and a seemingly endless parade of animal-free beverages.

Whichever prevails in the marketplace, one thing's for sure: While dairy producers tinker and tweak their product with state-of-the-art tech in efforts to make it more palatable to human digestive systems, more people than ever are looking at the concept of full-grown, supposedly weaned adults drinking something that comes out of an animal's teat, and calling it for what it is: Nuts!

Feb 5, 2015
Without Fish, Plenty More Food in the Sea

Have you heard? Science shows that, contrary to popular thinking, fish is not a vegetable.

Many so-called vegetarians harbor that fluid dietary ethic. I include my own 15 years as a so-called vegetarian, when I celebrated the occasional birthday or holiday with shrimp or New England clam chowder because, come on, "It's just seafood!"

But serious science has established a couple of other facts. One is that ocean drift nets grab a huge amount of "bycatch"—nontargeted animals that die just the same. By some estimates, that means a pound of other animals dying for every shrimp you eat.

We are emptying the oceans of sea animals; a recent study says that a quarter of species are threatened with extinction.

Sustainable, this ain't.

Additionally, in this century, scientific consensus has been reached on the question: Do fish feel pain? The answer is: Yes, these animals are sentient.

Luckily, science also has developed animal-free seafood options in all kinds of styles and formats. A new, tomato-based vegan sushi was detailed in a recent NPR story (1/23/15), and more everyday options are showing up at supermarkets.

"Vegan seafood—huh?" is the very appropriate tagline (considering how often I heard that when describing the topic of this month's column) for Sophie's Kitchen, which uses soy, pea and other vegetable proteins to create breaded "fish" fillets, "shrimp," "scallops" and "crab cakes" for the frozen aisle, plus Vegan Toona, sold in cans right next to the tuna fish at area Whole Foods stores.

I made a Toona sandwich—on toast, with vegan mayo—and it was tasty and satisfying, although I found tuna's signature smell muted.

Closer were the frozen, oven-ready, breaded options. The fillet, referencing milder fish such as sole, worked well with tartar sauce, as did the surprisingly convincing scallops.

The shrimp worked nicely with cocktail sauce. The pieces are shrimp-shaped, though without a crackly tail, and they have shrimp's slightly rubbery texture and even its red-on-white coloring.

Sophie's Kitchen has clearly tinkered for some time to achieve food that's reminiscent but not outright mimicry.

Another faux meat company, Gardein, has successfully forged ahead on the mimicry front. After making its name a few years ago with relatively easy-to-achieve chicken substitutes, Gardein upped its game with more difficult beef, and now, Fishless Fillets.

A blend of wheat, soy and pea protein, they continue the company's tradition of detailed quality. The crispy breading holds up very well and the "fish" inside is tender and tasty.

You also can make your own animal-free food of the sea.

Fish was never a personal fave for me, but I've missed that chowder, and not because of the clams. I found Isa Moskowitz's definitive New England Glam Chowder on the Post Punk Kitchen blog. (She now runs the vegan joint Modern Love, in Omaha, Neb.)

The chowder was terrific. Pureed cashews provided rich creaminess, with ocean flavor from ground-up sheets of nori seaweed. Coarsely chopped button and shiitake mushrooms stand in for the clams. ("Sea" for yourself at Philly.com/glamchowder.)

Though not as common as vegan beef or chicken, faux fish can be found in restaurants. New Harmony Vegetarian Restaurant has, since its plain old "Harmony" days, boasted a full vegan seafood menu. Vegan Commissary has an occasional fish-and-chips plate, and this month offers Nori Cakes, crab-cake-style patties topped with spicy, sun-dried tomato mayo in the platter version, or as a sandwich with Old Bay tartar sauce and hand-cut fries.

Allentown's Fresh Tofu makes Crabby Patties with vegan tartar sauce, sold fresh to-go at such outlets as Essene, in South Philly, Harry's Natural Foods, on Cottman Avenue in the Northeast, and Nature's Harvest, in Willow Grove.

The latter is, of course, where Horizons started. Some of us still recall Rich Landau's delicious tofu scallops. Today, his and wife Kate Jacoby's Vedge and V Street avoid animal-named items.

As an example, Landau mentioned the "beach style" Hon Shimeji mushroom stew from Vedge's opening days in 2011 (the recipe's in the *Vedge* cookbook from The Experiment).

It's not that the mushrooms are trying to imitate fish, he explained. "We can enjoy the beach flavors we might remember without harming sea creatures."

PERSONALITIES

Dec 11, 2014
Cory Booker Goes Vegan: "I Wasn't Living My Truth"

Cory Booker is known for blazing his own trail, jumping into the national spotlight as mayor of Newark, then winning a 2013 special election to become the first black U.S. senator from New Jersey.

Booker won a full term last month and, since that day, the vegetarian since 1992 has been conducting an "experiment" to eat strictly vegan for the rest of 2014.

After that, who knows? He could become the first vegan U.S. senator.

The day he tweeted his intentions was the same day that Center City vegan restaurant Vedge was named "Top Food" in Zagat's new Philadelphia Restaurant Survey. I tweeted that to Booker, which led to a Twitter conversation and the following phone chat (edited for space).

Q: So, have you encountered any interesting food situations since you've been eating vegan?

A: Thanksgiving was a big hurdle to get over. It's a holiday I thought of as macaroni and cheese, cornbread stuffing and the like. The fact that I was able to find such delicious, hearty vegan options that made me enjoy the holiday, I feel really happy about that.

The second thing is, there's a great vegan community out there—people who turn you on every day to a different food to try or places to go. In Washington, I tried the vegan gumbo at this one place, Eatonville, as an appetizer, and when all my friends were eating desserts—none of which were vegan—I just had another order of the gumbo. It was a wonderful experience.

Q: Do you cook at home? Any special favorites you could share with Daily News readers?

A: Well, I am no great cook, so that's a challenge. Tonight I'm gonna go home and steam some Brussels sprouts and peas. I'm gonna have a couple of vegan patties. It's very simple.

I've got a little bit of Vegenaise to put on it, or I have another type of mayonnaise, the Hampton Creek brand [Just Mayo] that's really good as well, so I'll put a little bit of that on it and some seasoning. I'm really looking forward to it.

Q: For as long as you've been vegetarian, the notion of going vegan must have occurred to you before. Why take the plunge now?

A: In 1993, I tried it for a while. It was a different time, and it just seemed incredibly hard. Everywhere I went, I had to say, 'Did you put butter on these vegetables?' I slipped back into a vegetarian lifestyle.

But the compelling reasons that made me become a vegetarian are pretty much the same compelling reasons for me to become a vegan. I almost felt like I'd been playing avoidance on [it] for a long time, just giving in to things like Ben and Jerry's and New Jersey pizza.

Q: You came into the Senate with a full plate of progressive causes. Is there any room to address animal agribusiness?

A: Absolutely. I'm very concerned about U.S. food policy. I posted a graphic yesterday comparing what our government says we should be eating—the My Plate, you know—and then you look at how we apply our subsidies. It's dramatically out of whack. We're subsidizing the very thing we tell people they should be eating less of.

If we're concerned about climate change as a country, we should have policies that make sure our great-grandchildren have a planet that's healthy and strong.

If we're concerned about high medical costs, we should have a government that's making sound investments with taxpayer dollars that don't contribute to the problem but actually help [solve] the problem.

Food is at the core of our lives in ways we don't always think about—how it affects our environment, how it affects our health and well-being, how it affects the expense of society, the expense of government.

Q: So, when 2014 ends, when, and how, will you decide whether to continue eating vegan?

A: One of the ideas I'm debating is going one more month, from Jan. 1 to Feb. 1, and inviting people to do a one-month experiment with me. Maybe do a video and see if we can get a lot of folks.

And we thought about reaching out to some existing vegan organizations to see if they would want to create a one-month trial with me and other folks.

I have to say, I feel a lot better, both emotionally and physically. And it's like simplifying your life.

While some people might think trying to be vegan would make your life more complicated, it's actually making my life more simple and cleaner.

I don't have that feeling of active avoidance. Like when you're rushing and you're in a hotel. I'd just order a plate of eggs—I found myself trying not to think about the origin story of those eggs.

When you find yourself trying to avoid the truth about something because it's inconvenient, because you know it doesn't align with your values and your moral compass . . . I wasn't living my truth. So, this has been a very good month, so far.

But also a strong part of me is, like, no judgment. I don't want to judge other people for their decisions. I'm a vegan who drives an SUV, for crying out loud.

Everybody struggles. We're all working to live our best selves, and we should do less judging and more encouraging.

Nov 10, 2009
Foer's Crusade: Famed Author Uses His Pen to Challenge Meaty Status Quo

Relax: For all his headline-grabbing talk about skinning and cooking dogs ["Let Them Eat Dog," *Wall Street Journal*, 10/31/2009], Jonathan Safran Foer doesn't want to challenge your values or change your mind about animals.

He does want to persuade you to stop eating factory-farmed meat. Not because it's against his beliefs, but because it's against yours.

That's the argument Foer, the author of *Everything Is Illuminated* (as well as *Extremely Loud and Incredibly Close*), develops in his new book, *Eating Animals* (Little, Brown and Co.). His "modest proposal" about dogs (including a recipe!) is a way of showing that we already know animals are individuals—we treat pets as persons, as members of our family—and he wants to make clear how thoroughly their lives are violated by factory farming.

Throughout the book, Foer details the commonplace animal suffering and misery in the system providing 99 percent of the meat and dairy we eat. He believes most Americans are still hazy firmly antithetical to what we're doing that it can just be a matter of time before it catches up."

Whether or not Foer's right, and MTV starts running "Say No to Factory Farming" PSAs any time soon, *Eating Animals* stands as a pop-cultural landmark, destined to be the starting point for a lot of overdue conversations.

Nov 21, 2013
A Meal Where Jews, Non-Jews and Turkeys All Give Thanks

A Thanksgiving dinner menu is already a complicated prospect. Add vegans (every extended family seems to have one), plus, this year, Hanukkah, and you might wonder whether it's even doable.

It is. Probably the highest-profile guidance can be found at the blog Kveller.com, by Mayim Bialik, star of TV's current hit "The Big Bang Theory" and formerly of "Blossom."

Bialik is an outspoken advocate of both veganism and Judaism, but it's her mother who's the T-Day host, sketching out and sending off an exhaustive (and happy-stickered) plan for a vegan "Thanksgivukkah" dinner that Bialik promptly posted on the blog with her own annotations.

In addition to Pumpkin Squash Kreplach and vegan chicken soup, the menu includes "One Large Rolled Gardein 'Bird,'" to which Bialik adds, "No friggin' clue how large it is, if it's shaped like a bird, and what it's rolled in or with."

Also on the menu, of course, are latkes.

"She was going to make another potato dish and serve baby latkes as the appetizer," Bialik told me in a phone interview from her Los Angeles home, but "I told her no, the only potato I think there should be on the table at Thanksgiving is a latke."

While her starch theory is strict, Bialik didn't have much to say about the "big protein" portion of the meal. "Honestly, if there's latkes, that's all my kids are going to eat, and that's fine."

There are also vegan sweets, of course.

"My mother requested that I make sufganiyot"—Hanukkah jelly doughnuts—"and I did hear that some people are filling them with cranberry jam, which I think is a great idea for Thanksgivukkah," Bialik chuckled. "But we happen to like them not filled, just with powdered sugar."

Watch for the recipe in *Mayim's Vegan Table,* a new cookbook coming from Da Capo this spring.

Whatever the dinner-table particulars, this confluence of cozy family holidays is a chance to amplify the gratitude inherent in each.

"We give thanks for the bounty of fruits, vegetables, grains, legumes and spices—all we need to thrive," said Jeffrey Cohan, executive director of Jewish Vegetarians of North America. "And as veg advocates, we are shining light in the dark places where farm animals are suffering."

Cohan noted that "the two themes of the combined holiday deeply resonate with us, as they should with all vegetarians and vegans."

One expert in holidays resonating through food is Nava Atlas, whose 2011 *Vegan Holiday Kitchen* (Sterling) veganizes many standard nonvegan dishes, grouped by their associated holiday. With a bounty of recipes for both Hanukkah and Thanksgiving, this collection is a trove of familiar dishes modified for all to enjoy.

Holiday dining should make everyone in your family—however you define it—feel welcome. Yet not every host, or guest, on how bad it is and need to grasp the scope of the problem. "It's not a question of needing to change anyone's values," he said by phone last week. "It's just making certain lines of sight clear, making connections."

Foer came to his newfound advocacy upon becoming a father. He and his wife had flirted with vegetarianism, always falling off the wagon. But now that he was responsible for someone's lifetime nutrition and health, Foer got serious about food and started researching its sources.

After sending repeated requests to well-known meat companies to visit their facilities—and receiving not a rejection, but no reply at all from anyone—Foer started looking deeper into the industry. Eventually his research led him to accompany an activist in breaking into a factory farm. What he saw and learned there helped turn him into a crusader.

As an already-celebrated author, Foer is positioned to shine a spotlight on common but little-known patterns and practices. He believes, for instance, that if more people were aware that all male chicks (around one out of every two chicks born) at big hatcheries are killed in terrible ways (including being thrown, alive, into a grinder), they would change their egg-buying habits.

But he knows not everyone who reads the book will go vegan, or even vegetarian.

"I think there are different respectable conclusions one can reach," he said. "What interests me most is mainstreaming the conversation in the same way environmentalism has been mainstreamed—making the question of what's at the end of our forks important, making the choice visible."

Foer noted that news since the book went to press has only bolstered his argument. A Worldwatch Institute study found animal agriculture to be a bigger contributor to greenhouse gases than all other factors combined. And new publicity about chicken feces in cow feed and veal calves being skinned alive has some looking more closely at the safety and ethics behind what they eat.

Add to that "the recent outbreaks of E. coli [two people dead, dozens sickened, half a million pounds of beef recalled by Fairbank Farms in Ashville, NY in early November 2009], the U.K. climate chief saying that the only way to save the planet is a movement toward vegetarianism—it's an argument that's unfortunately going to get stronger with time," Foer said.

But Foer knows people rarely abandon lifelong eating habits due to intellectual information, so he offers a compromise for meat junkies: Cut way down on your consumption (factory farming exists to meet Western consumers' outsize demand for meat at every meal), and eat animal products only from sources you know.

He profiles and reprints first-person narratives from several small farmers who are bucking the corporate trend and trying to provide their animals with healthy, humane lives before they're killed. Though in even these operations he finds trouble spots, Foer sees this as a trend worth supporting.

"Even if good [animal] farming is incredibly exceptional, to neglect it from the conversation is dishonest," Foer said. "And I'm interested in the kinds of change that are possible: It's impossible to imagine everyone in the world becoming vegetarian in this generation, but it is very possible to imagine factory farming being rejected."

Later in the conversation, Foer said he might have dismissed the everybody-vegetarian possibility "a little bit too casually" because "who'd have thought 20 years ago we'd have a black president? Or 10 or five years ago, for that matter? Some big changes come very quickly and I hope this is a big change that comes quickly."

While some animal-movement old-timers see in his proposals and optimism the naivety of a newbie, Foer is convinced that if enough eyes were opened to the facts, change would be imminent: "American values—not Democrat, not Republican, not liberal, not conservative, not urban, not rural, just American values—are so is an impassioned, skilled cook; some may be pushed out of their culinary comfort zone.

Bialik told me how her mother-in-law "had to make revisions to literally every single thing on the table" due to the prevalence of animal products.

Rachel Klein, of South Philly's Miss Rachel's Pantry, said she's lucky that "my Gran will make vegan latkes [without eggs]. But not everyone has that option."

Klein, an established catering and food-delivery maven, has a solution for hosts expecting vegans, or for vegan guests who want to bring something dazzling to the table. She's offering delicious individual meals and platters to share, too. "We've taken the traditional holiday protein and veggie sides and made them completely vegan so no one feels left out of the feast," she said.

Making the table a welcome place for all can be tricky, Bialik noted, "because there's this notion of what holidays 'have to be.'"

But there's a flip side, she added: "For those of us who value not eating animals, or the by-products of animals, we get to set a whole new set of traditions."

Mar 6, 2014
For Mayim Bialik, It's Vegan Parenting First, Neuroscience Second

Amy Farrah Fowler is a doctorate-holding neurobiologist on CBS's "The Big Bang Theory." Contrary to the saying "I'm not a doctor, but I play one on TV," actress Mayim Bialik, who plays Fowler, also has a doctorate in neuroscience.

Unlike Fowler, Bialik is also a mom, and a vegan one at that, two areas she's combined in a new cookbook, *Mayim's Vegan Table* (Da Capo). Written in a warm, easygoing, earth-mother style, the book addresses readers curious about vegan eating—for themselves but also, maybe, for their kids.

In a culture where stationing toddlers in front of a TV and buying them cheeseburgers at McDonald's is considered mainstream parenting, Bialik is already out of step. On top of her advocacy of natural childbirth, public breast-feeding and homeopathy, raising her two boys as vegans may seem outright kooky.

Vegan Table patiently but firmly straightens that out, building the case for a crunchy-granola lifestyle that does have crunchy granola but a lot more—peanut-butter smoothies, Brussels sprouts chips, vegan Reubens, oven-baked parsnip fries and chocolate-chip pumpkin cookies.

There's a lot of creative fun in the collection, as well as no-nonsense staples like potato salad, tomato soup, tacos and falafel.

For any readers still worried about the nutritional adequacy of plant-based eating at any age (attested to a decade ago by the Academy of Nutrition & Dietetics [known in 2003 as the American Dietetic Association]), Bialik was joined by pediatric nutritionist Dr. Jay Gordon to do what she called, in an email interview, the "heavy nutrition" for the book while she concentrated on more practical aspects.

"I'm just a mom," Bialik said, when I asked if her science degree helped with vitamin tracking. "I know a bit about biochemistry from my studies, and about brain development," but mainly, "I do my best as a mom who likes to be well-informed."

The book's recipes and advice are mostly drawn from first-hand parenting experiences and Bialik's quest to keep selections as healthy as possible while allowing for fun and, occasionally, junky foods.

"My sons are finicky. They like ketchup on everything," she said. "They do enjoy a variety of foods that many kids aren't exposed to. I try and get them to finish one bite of food before shoving another spoonful in, but I'm afraid I may be guilty of that sometimes, too!"

She said she's careful to avoid ultimatums centered on food. Parents may hang onto "a lot of fascinating ideas about what our kids 'should' eat," but sometimes "we need to recalibrate so our kids don't associate food with fighting and struggle."

Does she avoid conflicts with the "Mrs. Seinfeld" approach of hiding the healthy stuff?

"I don't sneak vegetables into things," she said. "I try and make foods that have vegetables prepared in enticing ways."

This may apply to such entries as Maple Mustard Greens and dilled chickpea burgers, which balance tasty fun with a nutritious punch. The book as a whole also strikes a balance: Bialik's "Mac N Cheez" is next to Sprout and Potato Croquettes with Dipping Sauce.

Also included are favorites from Jewish celebrations—hamantaschen, matzo-ball soup, sufganiyot, rugelach and more. The point here was more to offer good-tasting veganized versions rather than healthy them up.

In her teens, from 1990 to 1995, Bialik starred as the titular character on the TV show "Blossom." That's when she went vegetarian, "out of my love for animals."

Once in college, she cut her dairy intake way down "after having a lifetime of allergies. They virtually disappeared and I have not been on antibiotics or had a sinus infection since!"

She eliminated dairy and trace egg by the birth of her second son, after seeing her diet's effect on breast-feeding her children. She credits Jonathan Safran Foer's *Eating Animals* for inspiring the final kick.

Given her authorship of a book on the controversial practice of attachment parenting (2012's *Beyond the Sling* [Simon & Schuster]), Bialik might seem an easy target for skeptics of non-mainstream practices. When challenged, does she go into Amy Fowler mode, busting out the science and logic of veganism, or does she try to keep things intuitive and approachable, as she does in *Vegan Table?*

"I have no problem being very matter-of-fact about ethics and using a sense of humor to shake people up in a gentle way," she replied. "If pressed or challenged, I can pull out emotional arguments for sure, but I try to rely on logic, economics and the environment, with a touch of ethics, rather than going for the emotional jugular, as it were."

Whether working with kids or grown-ups, Bialik has both science and compassion on her side, and her cookbook demonstrates that she's prepared, whatever the occasion, to lay it all on the table.

May 7, 2015
Friends, Not Food
Farm Sanctuary's Gene Baur Sees His Humane Mission Take Root

Were you shocked to hear about Jon Stewart's post-"Daily-Show" plan to join his Philly-born wife, Tracey Stewart, in running a farm for rescued animals?

It was no surprise to Gene Baur, who has helped reshape attitudes—the Stewarts' and many others'—about food and animals since co-founding the first Farm Sanctuary for rescued farm animals almost 30 years ago.

Baur was a recent *Daily Show* guest, and when I inquired, post-interview, about reports that his first book, *Farm Sanctuary: Changing Hearts and Minds about Animals and Food* (Simon & Schuster, 2008), was a major influence on the Stewarts, he shrugged off the credit, saying, "All of us here at Farm Sanctuary are very grateful to the Stewarts." The couple will be honored in October at the Farm Sanctuary Gala at its home in Watkins Glen, NY.

Baur spent a good deal of his early years as an activist, along with sanctuary co-founder Lorri Houston, in and around Philly.

We talked by phone recently about Baur's advocacy approach and about his new book from Rodale, co-authored with Gene Stone, *Living the Farm Sanctuary Life: The Ultimate Guide to Eating Mindfully, Living Longer, and Feeling Better Every Day*. It contains 100 recipes, including one from Philly vegan restaurant Vedge. Here's an edited transcript of our conversation:

Q: This book features an impressive lineup of chefs. Did you have a favorite recipe?

A: (Laughs) Oh, no! That might be great, to pick the Philly one, Vedge. [But] I think they're all great.

Q: So have you been to Vedge?

A: I have not, but I am locked in on my calendar to be there the night before VegFest! I'm very excited about it.

Q: Is the spread of vegan eating going to encourage people to think in a big-picture vegan way?

A: Yes. There's a movement now in Philly and in other cities, too, to provide upscale and incredibly satisfying vegan cuisine. I think that's a big development. And then the vegan cheeses coming out. Miyoko Schinner's come up with some great ones, and other companies as well.

We like to think in a high-minded way about how people are going to behave according to their aspirations and values, and people want to do that. But realistically, the role of tasty, satisfying food is pretty important.

Q: What's your favorite food?

A: I have one of my recipes in the book, a special thing I do on weekends when I don't have to rush to be anywhere. I make scrambled tofu. Also, when I'm training—I've been doing marathons, and I did an Ironman Triathlon recently—I'm very focused on high-quality nutrition, so lots of greens, green smoothies.

I've been eating more fruits and vegetables—I really try to follow the Forks Over Knives recommendation.

Q: Your first book was a memoir. This one combines memoir, recipes and lifestyle how-to. Was that an intentional mix?

A: I think the new book reflects an evolution in our movement, actually. The first book was largely the history of Farm Sanctuary, a discussion of going into factory farms and more of a description of the problems with the animal-agriculture system.

This new book is for a broader audience and it's more of a how-to. It sort of assumes that people already have some general awareness of the problems of factory farming. It focuses more on what you, the reader, can do. It's really for everybody interested in living more mindfully, more healthfully and living in alignment with their own values.

Q: You were living in Wilmington when you started rescuing animals. Hilda, the famous first sheep, was found at a stockyard in Lancaster. Any particular memories from your time here?

A: The way we funded the organization in the early days was by selling veggie dogs at Grateful Dead shows out of our Volkswagen van. We spent a lot of time in the Spectrum parking lot, and I remember one time Pierre Robert, the [WMMR-FM] radio guy, came by and had a veggie dog.

Q: Establishing a farm sanctuary was a big step that others have followed. Did you see that as a way to change attitudes about food and animals, or just a way to help those that needed it?

A: A little of both. When we started in 1986, we didn't have a long-term vision of what the organization would be; we just responded to different needs in the moment. You find a [live] animal on a pile of dead animals, you take it home, you know, pretty soon you need more space so you get a farm. People want to visit, they want to hear about the animals, so you create a visitor program.

So, it's really been an evolution, and part of that is other people setting up sanctuaries, as well. I think that's a very positive sign. It shows people are re-evaluating our relationship with farm animals. This all boils down to our relationship with other animals: Is it based on respect or exploitation?

One thing that we have done, and others are doing it, too, is we model a different kind of relationship, one where the animals are our friends, not our food. Human beings like animals, and we tend to do what we see other people do. So, just doing this, I think, helped set an example that's now spreading.

Q: Do you worry about people seeing animals like this could think, "Oh, good thing they're not in a factory farm, I'll be sure to eat meat, milk and eggs from non-factory-farmed animals"?

A: We're very explicit about saying here the animals are our friends, not our food. If people see pictures put out by farms trying to sell this notion that animals can be raised and killed and consumed in a humane, respectful way—well, in my view, the words "humane" and "slaughter" do not sit well together. Often these labels that say animals are "treated humanely" or in a "free-range" situation sound a lot better than they really are.

Q: What's your next challenge?

A: We'll continue rescuing animals, educating people and advocating for reform to our food system. With the momentum of great vegan food, and also elite athletes talking about the benefits of plant-based eating, I think we're at a time now where there is a convergence of issues. I see us connecting more with environmental organizations, health organizations and other aligned interests and helping all that continue to expand.

Nov 5, 2015

Stewarts as Stewards

The Former Daily Show Star and His Wife Set to Provide Animals with Happy, Natural Lives Free of Fear

Jon Stewart's been much in the news of late, what with his new HBO production deal and the announcement that Farm Sanctuary's fourth animal-rescue enterprise will be at his and wife Tracey Stewart's 12-acre farm in Middletown, NJ.

That HBO deal is all Jon's, of course, but even casual observers know that Philly-born Tracey, a former veterinary technician, is in the driver's seat on the couple's animal-rights efforts. And there's more proof in her new book, *Do Unto Animals: A Friendly Guide to How Animals Live, and How We Can Make Their Lives Better* (Artisan).

Spanning genres with a one-of-a-kind mix of info, advice, philosophy and hands-on activities, the book also has some local biography: Stewart talks about growing up in Northeast Philadelphia and encountering her first dead bird while wandering the grounds outside a Bucks County carpet store where her parents were shopping.

Generally, though, the author keeps the focus on her subjects—all kinds of animals.

Do Unto Animals isn't a cookbook, but it does have recipes. How about the yummy-sounding oatmeal and molasses cookies on page 169? Sorry, they're not for you or me; they're to feed to horses.

"I am a terrible cook," Stewart confessed in an email conversation with the *Daily News,* "and that is why the recipes in the book are all for animals, whom I find to be a more forgiving audience."

And even though the book necessarily deals with food choices people make, it focuses on animals' individual interests. Chapters explain what makes a given animal happy, and what makes that same animal unhappy.

The tone throughout is good-humored and nonjudgmental, and Stewart paces herself carefully to avoid overwhelming the reader. She starts with house pets—the dogs and cats we know as individuals with needs and wants—then moves on to creatures we might encounter in the backyard, and then on to what makes cows, pigs and chickens unhappy. (Spoiler alert on the latter: It's being farmed.)

Stewart acknowledged working to meet readers where they are and ease them into the uncomfortable truths in animal farming, saying she was trying to "remind us that there are a never-ending amount of ways to [help animals]. I include just a small sampling of the horrors that animals face, because I know many loving and intelligent people that don't realize the magnitude of savagery that these poor creatures experience."

She points no fingers at those who, lacking information, may not yet be vegan. After all, "there have been many changes in myself over the years which included many different dietary choices. Along the way, I was still the same compassionate person I am today, whether I was eating meat or being vegetarian or vegan."

Still, she wants people to be able to make choices armed with real facts: "I know very smart people who assume that cows just always have milk and it's a relief for them when we come to milk them," she said, hitting on a tacit belief even I shared after 12 years as a vegetarian. She ran down the facts about forced impregnation, cows' maternal bonds and the immediate loss of their children (who would otherwise drink the milk the industry's based on), and how the males become veal.

"Knowing these things," she observed, "can move people to look for other alternatives that they otherwise might not have."

Stewart also spoke to the difference between small farm operations and sanctuaries, suggesting that we look beyond the green grass and sunshine: "An animal at a sanctuary receives individual care, medical attention and the promise of a full life. This promise isn't dependent on whether the animal provides something back. Even at the most 'humane' farms, you'll find that if an animal's medical care becomes counterproductive to profits, that animal will most likely continue to suffer or be 'culled.'"

On a sanctuary, animals "earn their keep" by being themselves. Stewart mentioned the pigs Anna and Maybelle as "the first ambassadors at our sanctuary," who already have a Facebook and Instagram following. "They are so funny and sweet!"

She encouraged readers to examine "what happens to the chickens at the farm where you buy your farm-fresh eggs when they start to lay fewer eggs or no longer lay eggs at all?

"For some individuals, the answer might not effect a change in them. However, others might then want to research further about what kinds of foods can be substitutes for eggs. In baking, mashed bananas can be used instead of eggs. That's a yummy fact to discover!"

So maybe Stewart does have some culinary chops. Is a cookbook next?

"If there is ever a *Do Unto Animals* cookbook," she vowed, "you can trust that there will be a co-author." But she seemed to warm to the concept: "It probably would be a great project for me to work on, because it would force me to learn to do better in the kitchen. My family would certainly appreciate that!"

As for her family, the Stewarts have two kids who are exploring dietary choices. But what about her husband, described in the book as a meat-eater? A recent *New York Times* piece brought up the reports that he's now vegetarian, and Tracey Stewart explained that "he's nervous about saying it publicly, because he doesn't want to mess up. But he really is trying to figure out what vegetarian foods he likes, and I'm helping him with that."

Be still our bleating hearts! Will the Jon Stewart who hits HBO in early 2016 be a new, improved, veganized version?

His wife was circumspect: "The best way to insure that someone will not become vegan is to try to convince them to be vegan. Live your own life, and hopefully your joy, and better health, will intrigue and inspire."

Exquisite vegan dining at a Philadelphia restaurant might also inspire, so how about a hometown trip? Stewart herself was shocked to report that "I have not been back since I graduated [from Drexel University in 1990]." But she's eager to try out what she aptly described as "a ton of fantastic vegan eateries awaiting me" here.

She stressed that her absence doesn't mean a lack of brotherly/sisterly love: "It's funny," she remarked, "whenever I meet someone else from Philadelphia, I immediately like them. Not only does Philadelphia make great soft pretzels, they make great people!"

Yeah! Tracey Stewart's husband isn't the only one who knows how to work an audience.

May 30, 2013
Eating Clockwise
Mark Bittman Has a Vegan-ish Idea—and It's about Time

Few food writers have done more to make vegans both cheer and grumble than Mark Bittman.

Certainly, the guy knows food, particularly the plant-based kind. He's a columnist for the *New York Times* Dining section and the lead food writer for the Sunday magazine. He writes for the Times opinion page and blogs, too. He also wrote the best-seller *How to Cook Everything* (Houghton Mifflin Harcourt, 1998)

Leafy greens are a trendy topic now, but Bittman wrote the book on 'em back in 1995 (*Leafy Greens,* Wiley). He's done a vegetarian cookbook and has examined some of the problems associated with overconsumption of meat.

Last July, he slammed the dairy industry, busting the ad claim that drinking milk prevents osteoporosis and sharing how his heartburn disappeared when he went milk-free.

But Bittman is neither vegan nor vegetarian, which frustrates many animal-free foodies who'd love to count the outspoken straight-shooter as one of our own.

With his new book, *VB6* (Clarkson Potter), Bittman pumps up that jam by suggesting that readers eat completely plant-based—until 6 p.m., when they can literally pig out. The book's full subtitle, "Eat Vegan Before 6:00 to Lose Weight and Restore Your Health ... for Good," marks its straightforward focus on health, although there's enough consideration of wider concerns to keep ethical vegans cheering—and grumbling.

When his doctor said to him, after some troubling blood work, "You should probably become a vegan," Bittman searched for a regimen that could improve his numbers and his weight while still allowing him to indulge in the foods he enjoyed most.

His only-after-6 approach isn't quite that simple, of course. The book could be called VUB6, because he also emphasizes unprocessed foods. It's not as though he's suggesting you eat Tofurky sausage for breakfast and Tofutti pizza for lunch, then fall "back" into an eat-everything dinner.

And even the B6 part has some wiggle room, as the plan is designed for individual customization. In an email exchange, I asked him how he went from one simple idea to a system whose kinks he'd worked out to the point that it was book-worthy.

"Really, I just started, plunged in without much of a clue," Bittman wrote back. "I believe any similar strategy that got me eating more plants and less other stuff would've worked. But this was easy and fine—after six weeks, I'd lost a bunch of weight and after 12 weeks my blood levels were all good. Both of those were stable for five years, and that's when I decided to write a book about it."

You can cheat here and there, and he does, but it's a sliding scale, he said. "To the extent I'm really strict about it, my weight stays down. When I cheat, it creeps up—which to me is a pretty good indication that it's sensible."

This positive-feedback loop helps make a plan like VB6 easier to adopt. Plus, many people find eating mostly whole, plant-based foods and less salt, sugar and dairy turns up your taste buds.

When I asked whether his palate had changed, Bittman wouldn't go that far, "but my satiety levels are different. I can make a stir-fry with very little meat or fish and think it's great. I really have adapted to the 'meat as treat' thing. I don't like dairy nearly as much as I used to, except good cheese. The rest of it I could take or leave."

VB6 indicts the high-fat, high-processed, high-meat standard American diet as a junk habit we need to break, Bittman said: "The science tells us we should be eating more vegetables and other unprocessed plant foods, and less of everything else. That is pretty much established. If you eat less junk and fewer animal products, and in place of those you eat plants, you're better off."

Bittman said he is presenting one strategy for doing that. "You can do it religiously, you can do it casually, or you can figure out another strategy: vegan except weekends, vegan after 9 a.m., vegan except Tuesday and Thursday—whatever. The idea is to shift the percentage of calories you get from unprocessed plants to as high a percentage as you can. Bearing in mind, again, that vegans eat junk food, too."

Fair enough. But couldn't similar results be achieved with an all-vegan plan that's unprocessed before 6, then pig out on vegan junk food after?

Sure, Bittman said.

So, if VB6 is good as far as it goes, why not go all the way? I was going to ask him, but Bittman had already answered that question in a blog post, "Why I'm Not a Vegan."

Some fans, he noted, had been grumbling, "Isn't being a part-time vegan like being a little bit pregnant?"

"Obviously not," he responded. To him, vegan means plant-based eating, which one can start, stop and restart at will. As for the 1944 Donald Watson definition—completely forgoing animal use—Bittman's not ready to go zero-hog, waiting for "the emerging dominance of a morality that asserts that we have no right to 'exploit' our fellow animals for our own benefit," or other trends that would make "universal, full-time veganism" a good blanket recommendation.

"VB6 is about changing your diet," he told me. "It's permanent and it's huge. Ethics enters into it, of course . . . we should not be torturing animals or treating them like widgets."

And then there's the planet: "Animal production as it stands now is probably the biggest agricultural threat to the environment," he noted.

VB6's health-motivation strategy could help people address these other issues by changing to more positive habits. "I'm more focused on real food than on pure veganism," Bittman said. "Junk food, highly processed food—animal or not—is really the biggest problem in health."

And if people cut down their meat and dairy intake, who'll complain? He reminded me that "any strategy that reduces animal consumption is a good thing."

Very true. And the more people eating animal-free for whatever reason, the more menus will adapt. Which leaves vegans like me with less to grumble about.

Grumble.

Aug 8, 2013
Neal Barnard's Book Is Full of Food for Thought

You might not call him a brainiac, but Dr. Neal Barnard is certainly brainy. He takes care of his gray matter and wants you to take care of yours.

Power Foods for the Brain (Hachette) is Barnard's latest book, and his thinking on food and health is worth paying attention to. Not just because he's a best-selling author, does nutrition research, teaches medicine at George Washington University School of Medicine and runs the nonprofit Physicians Committee for Responsible Medicine, all of which take mental acuity. It's more that he seems to think a decade or so ahead of the curve.

In addition to his own peer-reviewed research, Barnard points out trends among recent studies, pushing little-noticed issues into the mainstream conversation. Addictive junk food? *Breaking the Food Seduction: The Hidden Reasons behind Food Cravings—And 7 Steps to End Them Naturally* (St. Martin's Griffin) was on it 10 years ago. Genes that can be triggered, or not, by lifestyle factors? *Turn Off the Fat Genes: The Revolutionary Guide to Losing Weight* (Harmony) came out in 2001.

Power Foods covers brain-boosting foods but also threats, such as excess metals.

In a phone conversation, I asked Barnard if people should be "paranoid" about metal intake.

Well, yes, he said.

Iron and copper—meat's a big source of those—can be harmful when they oxidize in the brain, helping to release free radicals. Trace minerals are necessary nutrients, but whereas "you can eat a humongous amount of B6 or B12 without any adverse effects, with metals, if you tip even a little bit into excess, they can be harmful."

Daily multiple vitamins can be a concern, too, he said. "The vitamins themselves are fine, but the vitamin pill also includes metals that you don't need. So that's all part of the problem."

But if we go plant-based, I wondered, are we walking a tightrope to get the right amount of iron? Barnard assured me that there's a wide berth: "A vegan diet makes iron balance really easy."

In clinical research, people going animal-free for some health goal have found that their iron intake slightly increases, on average.

And it's all nonheme iron, "a form the body can absorb more of, if it needs more, or less if you're already in iron overload."

The heme iron that's in meat "tends to be too absorbable, so people tend to run into iron overload. And that's where you start talking about heart disease and Alzheimer's tied to iron excess," Barnard said.

Some fats can be a problem, but others are essential for quality brain work. Most of us have heard about the omega-3s in fish, though they're also available in plant foods. But how does one strike a perfect balance?

Barnard, a longtime advocate for vegan diets, said that the first key is to "get away from animal products. They're very high in the saturated fats that have been, in my view, clearly linked to Alzheimer's disease, but also to brain problems . . . earlier in life."

He pointed out that "around 8 percent of the calories in a typical green leafy vegetable are fat, and much of that is omega-3s." Maximizing those power foods while minimizing added fats (like those used in frying) will help achieve the best brain balance.

If you want to supplement, there are DHA supplements made with algae, so "you can go ahead and have that if you want," Barnard said, "but I don't think most people need them."

He also talked about brain-friendly (free radical-fighting) vitamin E, plentiful in seeds and nuts, though a lot of us overdo it with those, even the good doctor.

"If I buy a bag of cashews I guarantee you it's gonna be gone in about 10 minutes," he said. His portion-control tactic? Pour an ounce of nuts or seeds into the palm of your hand—"once it hits your fingers that's more than an ounce"—and crumble them onto salad, "as an ingredient, not as a snack."

Barnard also cautioned against relying on vitamin E supplements: "There are eight different forms of vitamin E in seeds and nuts, and they all have biological roles, but a pill has one or maybe two forms, and they tend to reduce the absorption of others from your diet."

As baby boomers age, mental decline and what can be done to forestall it is a growing issue.

"At the University of Cincinnati, researchers gave ordinary concord grape juice to people, their average age was 78 ... for three months they showed that it noticeably improved their memory and recall. They did the same thing with blueberry juice, same story."

Not that grapes and blueberries, which contain the anthocyanins that help learning and memory, are a magical antidote, but it can't hurt to bump them up in your eating routine. In another study, a brisk 40-minute walk three times a week was found to reverse natural brain shrinkage that occurs with aging.

Barnard is among a growing wave of doctors and scientists pushing for a bigger nutrition role in our health conversation.

There are still "a lot of folks like the smoker a generation ago, who knows that he or she should quit, but just isn't quite there yet," he said.

To help them along, he suggested experimenting with healthy, plant-based foods to find out what you like, then doing a three-week vegan test-drive.

After 21 days, "almost everybody is so delighted with it," he said, and "it's very easy to go forward at that point."

Barnard believes that we are in a place analogous to a generation ago, when doctors were themselves giving up smoking and getting serious about warning patients away from an established harm—cigarettes.

"Our generation," he said, "is doing the exact same thing with food."

Aug 10, 2015
Creator of *Earthlings* Looks at Bigger Picture in *Unity*

Vegans often hear that we should be paying attention to solving the problems of human society before worrying about the problems of animals.

I've shown that this is specious (as well as speciesist) given that the institutions humans have set up to exploit animals also invariably harm humans. But there's also a notion among vegans that mere avoidance of animal products should be only the start of more extensive good works.

In his new documentary, *Unity* (which opens August 12 nationwide), Shaun Monson paves some of that path, looking through a compassionate lens to show how our respect for animals and for each other are part of a whole, part of a positive system of relationships that we need to adopt—and soon.

Monson's previous documentary, *Earthlings,* is already legendary for presenting the issue of animal exploitation so clearly and powerfully that it has caused people to go vegan after the credits roll (I know people for whom this has happened), and has earned the moniker "the vegan-maker." Now Monson is using that cinematic method to treat a more mainstream issue. In a phone interview, he explained:

> "If you think about it, the press is always interested in [household] names, but they're also exceptional narrators. Particularly actors—they're very good with reading dialogue. In fact I

would've loved to have had a policeman or a janitor or a schoolteacher deliver those words, but actors know how to deliver that stuff the best and so I wanted actors. Even in *Earthlings* I worked with Joaquin Phoenix who was a vegan and an animal advocate, so that was pretty easy. This one was a little different—I didn't want it to be just animal advocates or humanitarians . . . [one film occurred with the other] and the idea was to see if they fit together in pieces as part of a whole."

So *Earthlings* and *Unity,* focusing on strife between humans and animals, and between humans and humans, respectively, will be part of a trilogy, of which the third part looks at humans and nature, in an ever-expanding sense of the whole. But the vegan idea still pervades the content as there's a parallel between our human "tribalism" that almost instinctively divides our family-and-friend group from other, more questionable humans, and the popular mantra "that's what separates us from the animals." As Monson put it:

"You can look at the history and see an attitude of empathy and compassion that is cultivated for the in-group, toward the family, the village, the nation, your favorite sports team, what have you, and in the same breath, while we're cultivating that empathy and love for the in-group, we're also cultivating an attitude of aggression toward the out-group, the other, and this is throughout the history of humanity. Animals aren't totally grouped outside of our group because we have many that live in our homes with us that families are fond of and consider family members, but in the movie we call it 'separation based on form' because we show empathy and compassion for some forms such as the dog, the cat, the whale, the dolphin or the harp seal, and in the same breath show an attitude of aggression toward other forms which might be the cow, the chicken and the pig. That's separation based on form, which I feel is mirrored in human society as well."

So will *Unity* turn out to be the "brotherly-love-maker"? I asked Monson if there was an analogy to going vegan that he was hoping to engender in viewers of this movie.

"I don't know that I have something that I want the viewer to do, because it should come from within—each person is different. But I do hope that we've shined a light on this ongoing contrast that seems to perpetuate itself continually in humanity, not just in our politics or our national conflicts but you even see it in our music, in our sports, in all of our stuff. In every film you can probably think of including Disney films you will see the 'princess' or the 'prince' and the 'evil king' or 'queen' are driving every story. The duality storyline is perpetually put forth, as if [humans] have one story that we know and it's presented the same every time. It's what we're being fed by constantly, so a new idea that's outside of that might seem sort of alien, or blunt, or radical, more philosophical, more spiritual . . . So yeah, they may come up with some new titles for what we have. I'm anxious to hear what they come up with."

Sep 3, 2015
Five Reasons the Pope Should Eat Vegan in Philly

Opinions are swirling about the pope's upcoming Philly visit for the World Meeting of Families—what will happen, what may happen, what should happen?

I have just one point: The pope should eat vegan while in Philadelphia. Here's why.

Reason #1. We want the pope to stay healthy. Pope Francis has made huge strides in bringing the papacy into the 21st century. But he's 78 and has spoken ominously about being called home early, and that's not what anyone wants. We're hoping for a John Paul II tenure (27 years, until he's 100).

Eating vegan may not be a cure-all, but a whole-foods, plant-based diet can reverse heart disease, and offers an array of health benefits. (The documentary *PlantPure Nation* goes into this in some detail.)

Kudos, then, to Aramark, which is supplying food to pope events. Aramark just announced a push for healthier food, with a greater emphasis on fruits and vegetables. Spokesperson David Freireich said that Sunday's Parkway event will include a vegan option—no exact details, but "largely produce-based."

Reason #2. The pope's not afraid to try new things. A lot of popes, frankly, were real sticks-in-the-mud about change. But this guy? First Jesuit pope, first "Francis," first Southern Hemisphere pope, first Western Hemisphere pope, first pope to tweet and first pope to have pizza delivered to him in his popemobile. For him, sampling Philly vegan fare is a piece of cake (especially if he stops by Sweet Freedom on South Street.)

Why not first vegan pope, too? It would fit right in.

Reason #3. He's a bridge builder. Rather than stick with a parochial notion of spirituality, this pope has sought common ground, both within his own faith (the Orthodox churches) and across the aisle (he's celebrated his strong Jewish ties with acts such as officially observing Rosh Hashanah). Calling for more interreligious dialogue, he's actually used the term "building bridges."

Thing is, the avoidance of animal products is common to ancient (and some modern) versions of many religious disciplines. Some sacred Catholic days call for vegan or near-vegan eating. Both

Hebrew and Muslim law spotlight the avoidance of different animal products—Hindu, too.

Skip all animal products, and the pope instantly builds a bridge.

That cross-cultural impulse is easy in our town, whose oldest vegan restaurant, New Harmony, in Chinatown, is also certified kosher. So is one of the newest, Miss Rachel's Pantry, in South Philly. Kosher-certified VGE, in Bryn Mawr, is just a couple of towns away from St. Charles Borromeo Seminary, where Pope Francis will be based. Near-vegan venues Mama's Vegetarian (100 percent kosher) and Govinda's (Hare Krishna) also offer a wide variety of spiritually nourishing foods that easily cross borders, while tasting great.

And, though everyone will direct the pope to a favorite haunt for a cheesesteak, kosher-certified Blackbird Pizzeria has the definitive item—plus incredible vegan varieties of that current papal favorite, pizza!

Reason #4. He named himself after the patron saint of animals. Saint Francis of Assisi famously preached to birds and said of animals that "not to hurt our humble brethren is our first duty" and that our next is "to be of service to them wherever they require it." Taking the pope's namesake at his word means being vegan, as animal foods can't be produced without hurting them.

It must be pointed out, though, that the evidence that Saint Francis himself lived by this ideal is scant.

Pope Francis's encyclical, *Laudato sí,* garnered headlines for talking about climate change. But it also stated that "it is contrary to human dignity to cause animals to suffer or die needlessly." Pope Francis repeatedly called for a new balancing of animals' interests with those of humans and declared obsolete the concept "that other creatures are completely subordinated to the good of human beings, as if they have no worth in themselves and can be treated as we wish," and he condemned as non-Biblical "a tyrannical anthropocentrism unconcerned for other creatures."

In other words, thinking of animals as tools and property to be used and exploited needlessly is archaic and should be abandoned. OK, good point—all that remains is to live it!

Reason #5. Really? Travel 4,358 miles to Philadelphia and miss Vedge?

Let's cut to the chase, Your Holiness. Vedge isn't just the restaurant with the best food in Philly (according to 5,000 Zagat survey respondents). It's also, in the words of one globetrotting vegan journalist, "possibly the best vegan restaurant anywhere." And its owners, Rich Landau and Kate Jacoby have already prepped two perfect dishes for your meal, as teased out by Marilyn D'Angelo at *NewsWorks*.

Landau generated an eggplant braciole that fits with the cuisine of central Italy, combined with a Sicilian salsa verde, while Jacoby offered potato pierogies with a Latin twist.

Obviously, you don't have to stick to these custom creations; everything at Vedge is fantastically fitting for the palate of the top prelate on the planet.

Now, I realize *il papa* is a man of simple tastes, who might prefer to spend all day sipping Yerba mate (which you can get at Grindcore House cafe!) or chomping on a soft pretzel (not all are vegan, but Center City Pretzel Company's are).

Still, you should take some time out to visit Vedge and encounter food that's fun, forward-looking and dedicated to peace and fairness, much like your own pontificate.

You may think I'm exaggerating. But one bite will make you a believer.

VEGAN IN THE WORLD

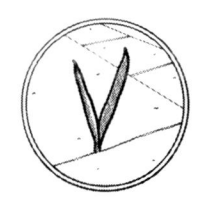

Aug 22, 2013
Past Presidents' Precedents for Veganism
Founding Fathers Feasted on More than Meat, as Some Eateries Prove

The olden times, they are a-changin'.

Last week, the dinner-theater chain Medieval Times, which specializes in meaty, sometimes cheesy "royal feasts," announced a 30th-anniversary upgrade: the addition of a vegan menu.

As wild as that is, it turns out this is just one of many history-based dinner providers, national and Philly-based, that are adding veggie menu options to their repertoire—and in some cases, not even compromising on historical authenticity.

At the best-known historical-immersion destination, Virginia's Colonial Williamsburg, menus have been "traditional" since the town was relaunched as a tourist destination in the early 1930s. But last year, one of the town's signature historical restaurants introduced a vegan burger to its dinner menu.

I wanted a firsthand look-see.

On a family vacation—and my first big road trip in a while—I was gratified to find that traveling vegan is getting easier. Let me give a shout-out to two prime examples: The Richmond, VA, veggie spot Fresca on Addison had great vegan sandwiches and desserts, and the irrepressible Bob Tubbs at The Cedars of Williamsburg B&B had vegan pancakes and much more at the ready from the first breakfast.

The Williamsburg restaurant in question is Traditions, in the Lodge, where executive chef Rhys Lewis and chef Justin Addison developed the new burger, a blend of navy beans and black-eyed peas. With the usual fixins but sandwiched between flat pitas, this is a concoction both singular and tasty, with a solid spice blend that gives the beans a kick.

Addison explained that the idea for the burger came while picking (historically correct) navy beans at a local farm. But this may be just the start—Addison looked forward to eventually doing "something different for vegans and vegetarians every day."

Meanwhile, back in Old City, historical mainstay City Tavern last year introduced fried tofu as an entrée, supplementing vegan appetizers and sides like potato leek soup and corn chowder.

Wait, tofu? In Colonial Philadelphia? It turns out Benjamin Franklin (who tried vegetarianism on more than one occasion) sent a 1770 letter to John Bartram including instructions for making an animal-free cheese called "tau-fu" from "Chinese caravances" (soybeans). Yes, independence wasn't the only campaign of which old Ben was an early adopter.

City Tavern owner and executive chef Walter Staib said adding a tofu entrée was "one of the best decisions I ever made," as the dish has wound up "a top seller" at City Tavern.

The straight-off-the-menu version is vegetarian, but is breaded with egg and served on linguine that also has egg; the vegan alternative—which Staib noted "tastes just as good"—is a broiled tofu served on a bed of seasonal veggies.

Was it the letter that inspired the addition, or was that a convenient excuse to diversify the menu? Staib allowed that "I was getting a lot of requests for vegetarian options," and having researched the Franklin tofu issue, he decided the time was right to do something tasty with the information.

So is this vegging up of historical menus stretching the notion of "authentic" to fit modern tastes and health concerns?

Not necessarily, Staib said. "In the 18th century, a lot of people were vegan [i.e. plant-based eaters] not by choice, but by circumstance."

Addison concurred: In Colonial times, "there were a lot more vegetables and a lot more starches served" than present-day menus might indicate.

Even among those who had the means to feast on flesh, some intentionally cut back. Thomas Jefferson, a prodigious gardener, said he ate meat only "as a condiment to the vegetables which constitute my principal diet."

In the context of the times, he was a "near-vegan," said Staib.

So Franklin wasn't the only culinary visionary in Independence Hall. And as it happens, Jefferson was also mentioned as inspiration by Justin Addison, who noted that "Chef Rhys and I are eating more like that these days."

In fact, Traditions should have "an entire vegetarian and vegan menu" as early as next year.

All that Colonial-era reminiscing, and the pitching of independence to the man in the dirt street, got me musing: Just as explicit human rights slowly dawned on the popular mind in the face of traditional might-makes-right colonialism, might the logic of sentient-animal justice be slowly dawning on traditional might-makes-right "carnivore" foodies?

Too early to tell, but as we move forward, there's one thing you can count on.

"You're going to see more vegan restaurants," Staib predicted. "I think it's here to stay."

May 29, 2014
Elbows without Grease
V Is for "Veg" as Much as for "Violent" among Local Roller Derby Jammers

Plant-based foods: Powerful enough to knock you on your ass?

Indeed. Especially as processed by some Philly Roller Girls who fuel themselves with "kinder, gentler" foods as they elbow their way to the top of their tough game.

Our Delaware Valley league has around 50 women on four teams, including the Liberty Belles all-stars. More than a dozen PRG members are vegetarian and/or vegan-leaning eaters, estimated league spokeswoman Erica Vanstone.

That's a high ratio. How come?

I've been wondering since 2011, when I heard of PRG's support for Little Baby's vegan ice cream flavors. Later, I would often run across a PRG connection at veg-friendly events I covered, such as the Vegan Wing Bowl.

When Blackbird Pizzeria grabbed the decisive lead in the *Daily News* Vegan Cheesesteak Contest earlier this year, after a 30-strong PRG "NoshMob" voted for the place while eating there, I knew I had to investigate.

First, let's get up to skating speed: The Philly Roller Girls formed in 2005 as part of a resurgence in interest in a contact sport that got its start in the '30s.

These days, skaters play on a flat track instead of the banked tracks of yesteryear that you may recall from TV broadcasts. The latter also imposed pro-wrestling-style story lines, while the current version's simple theme is women pushing themselves to their full potential.

The emphasis on athletics over theater has made the amateur sport, governed by the Women's Flat Track Derby Association, very competitive. Vegan fuel provides the edge that some players want while reflecting inclusive derby values.

Three Philly all-star players are 100 percent plant-based: Angela Luczejko (Antidote), Mishel Castro (Castro) and Caroline Voyles (ClamJammer). They're among "the most competitive and talented in our league," Vanstone said, adding that since PRG is one of the top 20 leagues worldwide, they really are "some of the best players in the world."

And "you'd never pick them out of a lineup as vegan," she said.

When I stopped by a practice in Camden to meet them, Castro picked up on that theme.

"Any time you mention you're vegan, someone's like, 'What do you do for protein?' Like you're about to wither away and die," she said, laughing. "They see us out there [skating] and they're like, 'Hmmm, you're actually really muscular for your size—and you're vegan?'"

While the old-timey notion of weakling vegans has been exploded over the years by vegan boxers, ultramarathoners, pro football players, Olympic medalists and the like, some people haven't gotten the memo yet. But there's another oddity: Given its tough attitude and rough contact, is roller derby consistent with a compassionate diet?

"Sure, it's a 'violent' sport," admitted ClamJammer, "but it's also something not violent—it's empowering to be strong and to be women [pursuing] a goal. Now, if vegans are supposed to be peaceful and quiet..."

She broke off with a "can't help ya" look, as the others agreed that Derby and veganism dovetail.

"It's such a nontraditional sport—for people who are already kind of breaking out of boxes for whatever reason, so it may be easier to go, 'Yeah, let's give [veganism] a whirl, too,'" ClamJammer explained. "Roller derby is really welcoming to a lot of people—there's no stereotypes. We're all here."

Antidote, a longtime vegetarian, went vegan late last year after surgery for an on-track injury.

"I spent a lot of time researching vegan athletes," she said. "I was finding bodybuilders and MMA and kickboxers, and I really found almost a spiritual side of it—the clean food—because everything you eat becomes part of you. The more I want to compete, the cleaner I want to eat."

Castro has been a force in moving the group overall in a more veg-friendly direction. "I've been involved with managing our travel all-stars for many years," she said. When she started scheduling lunches at Whole Foods, "they were like, 'I'm not eating this healthy crap.' But . . . now the team is completely on board."

Roller Derby appeals to "people from all walks of life," said Vanstone, so "it's a place where ideas cross-pollinate frequently." She oversees frequent PRG outreach events suggested by members.

The Vegan Wing Bowl at The Abbaye in Northern Liberties was Vanstone's idea "because I used to work there and thought PRG was a great fit."

Skaters have found that vegan eating fits for diverse reasons.

ClamJammer focused on ethics: "Environmentalism and the welfare of animals are a big motivator for what I choose to eat."

Castro has found cleaner eating to be a necessity: "I can't put crap in my body as fuel to be one of the best players on the team anymore." Though on the flip side, she added, "I'm getting older and I'm still not putting on weight 'cause I eat awesomely."

Antidote said that, for her, vegan eating "fell into place" since she's lactose intolerant and "just never liked the taste of meat."

The inclusive awareness plays out in the sport, said Vanstone: "For out-of-town tournaments, wherever you go, the welcome package will feature a vegetarian or vegan item. And we're always conscious of vegetarian and vegan eaters who attend our events."

To wit: Little Baby's will bring its vegan flavors to Saturday's bout.

ClamJammer opined that "in terms of a fan base, too, people who are more open-minded about their sports-watching and might go see 'that weird thing on roller skates,' they might also be more willing" to try foods that are outside the mainstream.

*

The Right Track: Soup, Shakes . . . and Peanut Butter

Philly Roller Girl all-stars Angela Luczejko (Antidote), Mishel Castro (Castro) and Caroline Voyles (ClamJammer) stress that their diets vary dramatically in season and off. I asked about the foods they associated with derby days. Here are their responses, edited for space.

Antidote

I eat a lot of raw food—nuts and seeds, you know—and a lot of Asian food. I love sushi, love avocado rolls and especially sweet potato rolls. I have sushi at least once a week.

I tend to do five small meals a day. I'll have soup in the morning or afternoon—mushroom soup on a consistent basis. Usually a protein shake with different kinds of berries in it. Orange juice in it a lot of the time. Eating out, the Caesar salad at Blackbird [vegan pizzeria on 6th Street] is good.

After a game, though, the instant I'm all unguarded, it's "Where's my root beer?"

It's cold, refreshing and I don't drink it normally, so it's like a treat, and it gives me quick sugar in my system. So that maybe once a week, and also Justin's peanut-butter cups. The dark chocolate ones are vegan.

Castro

I don't know if you've heard of Vega—they're plant-based vegan sports supplements, more or less. So I usually have a protein shake after I skate.

On a day of a game, I eat the amount of food that would feed a small family somewhere. I don't like to eat a couple of hours before the game, so I pretty much wake up and put everything I own in my face: Tofu scramble with coconut pancakes is my favorite, and then I'll have oatmeal with a banana, and then I'll probably have quinoa, and then I'll probably make a shake.

That's the best part—I love to eat. I'm Italian [so] my family thinks I'm crazy for the kind of diet I have, but, to be honest, it means that I can eat what I want all the time. And more often than not, it's awesome.

ClamJammer

My favorite thing is peanut butter. Yeah, I've tried to do almond butter, but it gets so expensive—I eat too much of it.

Peanut butter is . . . if you're sitting in a rink all day and the concession stand has hot dogs and nachos, you're not gonna be getting any of that, so peanut butter and banana became the easy thing to bring. And it's protein, and so I do that a lot.

In terms of a daily regimen, I do not want to eat anything three hours before [a game], so I'll have oatmeal with peanut butter and bananas and other good stuff in it, or maybe a quinoa porridge if we're not on the road. Some fruit here and there, with peanut butter on it, of course, and then take a break.

After a game, I can't eat anything right away, maybe some Powerade, you know, something sugary. And then . . . yeah! More peanut butter!

Nov 3, 2011
On a Tight Budget? Lose That Pricey Meat

Whatever you think about Occupy Wall Street and Occupy Philly, there's now a lot more discussion about economic inequality and the struggle of many to put food on the table.

Food economics is key in downtown Philadelphia, too, as the protesters, with the help of their allies, provide three meals a day for anybody who shows up hungry. Notably, a lot of those meals are vegan.

It's not so much from a commitment to nonviolence or to boycott a corporate-dominated agricultural sector. The main reason is that plant-based food is cheap and easy to make—a boon to a built-from-scratch operation like Occupy.

Peanut-butter-and-jelly sandwiches are always on the menu, but there are also hot meals, thanks to groups like Hare Krishna, whose vegetarianism is part of their mission, and the Quaker Friends Center.

"I would say almost all the meals here have at least had a vegan option. Most meals are vegetarian, at least, and a lot have been vegan," said "Kevin," an Occupier who has assisted in some meals. "A lot of the donations like canned goods just happen to be vegan. Meat is pretty rare because we have no way to store it to keep it at a proper temperature for health reasons."

At home, you likely have a way to regulate food temperature. But using less meat can help stretch a food budget. A recent study in the *American Journal of Clinical Nutrition* said a good way to save money while improving health is to replace "some red meat with less-expensive whole grains and beans."

Last year, prolific cookbook author Robin Robertson released *Vegan on the Cheap* (Wiley), with "pennies-a-serving" recipes and tips such as checking ethnic groceries for staples and making your own condiments.

Robertson points out that if you have a yard, or just a windowsill, you can grow some of your own food, another plant advantage.

This year saw the more specific *Eat Vegan on $4 a Day* by Ellen Jaffe Jones (Book Publishing Co.), a former TV investigative reporter. She goes into the consumer-rip-off aspects of our food system, such as the Department of Agriculture spending to promote meat and dairy vs. fruits and vegetables. *Eat Vegan* also has tips and recipes.

Four dollars a day too extravagant? The blog series "Vegan for $3.33 a Day" chronicles how one woman puts these ideas into practice with even more savings.

How low can these plant-strong penny-pinchers go? A dollar a day is a nice round figure—anybody?

The lower on the food chain you eat, the lower your risk of disease and the better for the environment. In other words, going veg-based can be easy on your wallet and "low-cost" to the planet. Moreover, it addresses the biggest imbalance of all: The oppression of animals.

After all, the ratio of human to "food animal" life lost is 1 to 1,000. Talk about being among the 99.9 percent—and a dead-end job!

Not one of us can rid the world of injustice. But all of us can strive to rid our plates of it.

Feb 9, 2012
Vegetarian + Love: Can Couples Make It Work?

It's always the same old story: Boy meets girl . . . or boy; girl meets boy . . . or girl . . . Anyway, the part that's the same is that two people come together from divergent worlds and try to turn those two worlds into one.

Whether they hit it off depends on a lot of factors, and one of the biggest—and hardest to ignore—is food. All of us have foods we like or dislike, of course, but when one would-be lover is a vegetarian or vegan, and the other isn't, the issue is much more pronounced.

Will somebody switch sides? Will they create a separate-but-equal dinner detente? Will they compromise in little steps, trying to reach a general consensus?

There are probably as many answers as veggie/non-veggie couples. Sure, some so-called "vegansexuals" draw a hard line, with a mantra of "Lips That Touch Liver Will Never Touch Mine." Others prefer to jump into the fray, mix it up and see what happens.

South Jersey's Anne Dinshah is one of those adventurous souls. You could say she wrote the book on this topic, because she did. It's due out at the end of this month.

Dating Vegans (American Vegan Society) grew from Dinshah's column in *American Vegan* magazine and is largely a chronicle of her matchups over one dedicated year with men, some of whom were not quite vegan, and others who were wayyy not vegan. She talks about how they reacted to her veganism and what foods they found as common ground. She even interviews her exes to get their take.

One ex, Brad Holdren, told her, "On the grand scale of 'squeezing the toothpaste' issues, vegan is not huge. Other topics, like kids or religion, seem tougher. I gotta believe it's just a learning process that involves cooperating together."

Across the board, Dinshah said, "what worked best was asking a guy what are his three favorite vegetables, then I would craft a delicious entrée using those."

Sometimes she worked the other way, though. "One guy dared me to make him like Brussels sprouts. I made him three dishes and he like all of them, including a fruit pie that has Brussels sprouts in it!

"It always impresses a man if you can make a dessert he likes," she added. "Everybody likes dessert."

The book includes recipes for treats like easy vegan fudge and almost-as-easy brownies (see recipes at Philly.com/veganchoc) that even those who are not as handy in the kitchen can make. "If you really want her," Dinshah advised male readers, "make her some chocolate. You're going against the stereotype."

There are also perspectives from couples who have come up with their own solutions to the "food compatibility" issue. These make *Dating Vegans* a wider resource for anyone who has an interest in love, as the methods of resolving these differences spill out into other issues couples face.

But no matter who you are, Dinshah said, love comes down to "chemistry and compatibility: You need both. Opposites attract, but not too much! There has to be an overlap, an intersection, and food is always part of that."

Mar 5, 2015
Will New Dietary Guidelines Survive Big Meat's Ire?

"New diet guidelines: a death knell for meat-eating?"

Headlines for February's long-awaited Dietary Guidelines Advisory Committee recommendations practically shouted as much.

And the meat industry seemed to agree: Barry Carpenter, president and CEO of the North American Meat Institute, quickly slammed the committee for a "flawed" report "generalizing about an entire category of foods," although that's exactly what the guidelines have done since back in the "Four Food Groups" days.

At issue is a shift in the overall favorability of flesh-based foods in the diet: When the guidelines were last revised, in 2010, they said that healthy eating "emphasizes . . . lean meats and poultry," while the new recommendations would say a healthy diet is "lower in red and processed meat."

Scooting meat over the line from mildly positive to mildly negative is a strong move, but one that Dr. Michael Greger, who runs NutritionFacts.org, expects to see diluted when the official guidelines are released. That could come later this year, but there's no guarantee.

That's because the meat industry (and sugar interests, too, since sugar also took an unprecedented hit) will be lobbying tirelessly to influence the final product, as they did when the four food groups (half of which were animal products) gave way to the food pyramid in 1991.

That changeover was delayed for a full year by industry battles. The official Dietary Guidelines for Americans are updated every five years, while the iconography changes sporadically. (The pyramid was replaced by MyPlate in 2011.)

Greger, who testified before the committee, also addressed the easing of warnings on dietary cholesterol, which garnered wild-eyed headlines telling Americans that eggs are now a health food. Greger explained that, given the amount of animal foods in the standard American diet, we can "max out the ability to absorb dietary cholesterol." After that, additional amounts don't make much difference.

"If you throw a lit match into an already blazing puddle of gasoline, it doesn't seem to have much of an effect," he observed. "But cut out all [dietary] cholesterol, and you'll see a great difference.

"When it comes to cholesterol [in the blood], which we know to be part of the disease process," he said, the equation is not that complicated: "Whatever food increases it is a bad thing, and any food containing fiber will lower it."

Part of the shift against meat in the proposed guidelines comes from factoring in "sustainability," since animal agriculture is extremely resource-intensive. But I find that a mixed bag.

Sure, destroying the planet is ultimately bad for our health, but people are already looking for an excuse to ignore the guidelines and eat whatever they want, and external issues like climate change just play into that impulse.

When I railed about this to Greger, he countered that such a wider scope is not unprecedented, citing the '70s-era guidelines' advice to lower alcohol intake, not so much due to immediate health effects as to its factoring into fatal car accidents. Fair enough.

While meat takes heat in the advisory committee's recommendations, some experts question the continued emphasis on cow's milk, a common childhood allergen that also causes digestive problems for most adults.

Last fall, a large Swedish study involving over 100,000 people followed over 20 years ("Milk intake and risk of mortality and fractures in women and men: Cohort studies," *BMJ 2014;349:g6015*) found scant evidence for milk protecting bones, reinforcing previous studies showing no such correlation. The study instead found a stronger association between milk-drinking and mortality.

In short, the cute "Dairy" cup shoehorned into the USDA's current MyPlate graphic looks like an elective add-on that tells us more about corporate interests and inertia than about Americans' diet needs. It may be 2020 before we can see that as clearly as we do the meat group.

These are my reactions to the report; yours may well be different. Public commenting is open at health.gov/dietaryguidelines/dga2015/comments/ through April 8, 2015.

May 2, 2013
Veganism: The "Whole" Picture

If I say "vegan rock star," Chrissie Hynde or Moby or Jason Mraz might come to mind. You wouldn't immediately think of T. Colin Campbell, 79, professor emeritus of nutritional biochemistry at Cornell University.

But Campbell's half-century of research in nutrition, hundreds of peer-reviewed papers and a key role in the world's most comprehensive study of health and nutrition, the "China Study," have surely made him a rock star in the plant-eating world.

He summarized that groundbreaking study (which the *New York Times* called "the Grand Prix of epidemiology") in a 2004 book of the same name, co-authored with his son Thomas. He co-starred in the documentary *Forks Over Knives,* and was part of the team that helped Bill Clinton go plant-based. So there's plenty of anticipation for his new book, *Whole* (BenBella), out this week.

A "whole-foods, plant-based" (Campbell introduced the "WFPB" term at a National Institutes of Health panel in 1978) eating pattern is the most scientifically sound approach for optimum health, he asserts, noting that plants offer unique antioxidant benefits while, conversely, animal protein is associated with a wealth of disease risks.

Campbell wishes that more people understood the basic science showing the WFPB benefit.

"If you took the best of medicine, it cannot match what this can do," he said in a phone interview. He faults an emphasis on reductionism—red wine is good for you in this study, bad for you in another—for sowing nutrition confusion among the public.

Having started his inquiry as a dairy farmer looking to maximize yields, Campbell for many years "worked and researched on a nutrient-by-nutrient basis," but has come to see nutrition as "multiple mechanisms acting in concert."

Far from an animal-rights idealist, Campbell went vegan on the basis of the evidence.

With decades of data and food-policy experience under his belt, Campbell speaks candidly and lets the chips fall where they may—even if it's in the compost heap.

Here's the kicker for self-satisfied vegans touting the meat-vs.-plants stuff: The optimal WFPB plan excludes all oil, all added fats.

Come a-whaaaa? *Who is this crackpot?*

French fries? Onion rings? Margarine? "Heart-healthy" olive oil? *Zero?* Seriously?

Seriously.

Campbell's medical colleague Caldwell Esselstyn succeeded in reversing heart disease in patients with an animal- and oil-free eating plan. This stricter regimen also appears effective at fighting weight gain, diabetes and cancer.

But come on, how can Joe Average live without oily food?

Fortunately, along with *Whole*, BenBella is releasing *The China Study Cookbook*, showing how healthy WFPB meals can be delicious and simple to prepare.

There seems to be an entire spring campaign pushing WFPB, with May also seeing the release of Rip Esselstyn's *My Beef with Meat* (Grand Central). The younger Esselstyn (Caldwell's son) was an Austin, TX, firefighter/EMT who got his whole firehouse to go WFPB with terrific results. He too is something of a vegan rock star, and in this book he delivers not just facts about the livestock industry but 140 WFPB recipes.

Probably the most established and popular cookbook chef in this field, though, is Lindsay Nixon, whose *Happy Herbivore* books have brought the WFPB ethos to millions, with added doses of fun and creativity. She recently released *Happy Herbivore Abroad* (BenBella) and is now working on her fifth book in the series.

Whole is a welcome volume—a rock-star follow-up that avoids the sophomore slump—but even if you don't want all the backstory, you can start with one of the recipe books and try these healthful dishes for yourself.

You have nothing to lose but your food chains!

*

Interview with T. Colin Campbell, Author of *Whole*

V for Veg: What's the key difference between The China Study *and* Whole? *Why did you feel the need to follow-up?*

T. Colin Campbell: *The China Study* was basically a summary of the evidence and what I thought it showed. It was based on my own career, of course, but also involving the work of others. *Whole*, in contrast, is to count why.

In other words, *The China Study* was: Here's the scene, here's the evidence, here's what we think it says. And *Whole* is sort of an explanation of why this evidence actually works. It really has a dramatic effect on health—even more than I thought when I finished writing *The China Study*. I mean I was pretty confident in what I was saying, of course, but nonetheless, since that book was published, what we now know about this is just truly dramatic.

V for Veg: Are the beneficial effects of the whole-foods, plant-based diet more ascribable to the positive effects of the plant foods or to the elimination of animal protein's liabilities? Which one has the greater impact?

T. Colin Campbell: Well, I don't particularly care for trying to describe things in quantitative estimates of things. That often leads to a lot of controversy and dispute over the numbers, so I don't like to do it that way.

Let me explain it this way: What I had attempted to do after my four-plus decades of research was to try to reconcile all the details that people talked about involving the relationship between diet and health and so I assembled some of the detailed evidence and tried to synthesize an idea, and that idea was that a whole-foods, plant-based diet has the most potential for offering good health. And it turns out it works . . . and that, as you may recall, was the opposite of what I thought might be true when I started my career some 40 years before—I had come from a dairy farm, I had covered the science, I had worked and researched on a nutrient-by-nutrient basis and learned all those years . . . and so we tried to knit together the details. That's what we tried to do, with my son who co-authored the book with me—he's now a physician, by the way, he was an actor in Chicago later, I had gotten him to help me write the book but in the process he became enthused about this idea, went back to medical school he's just now finishing up his residency and he lectures himself now—in any case, we knitted together this story that I thought made sense, and as I say, it really works on a broad spectrum of different kinds of diseases and it works very quickly, the most benefit, [more] than anything else in medicine. If you took the best of medicine, it cannot match what this can do.

So I got very excited about it, very optimistic about it, and then I thought, well, how come we've gotten it so wrong? When I say "we," I'm talking about my community of research as well as the clinical practice community—basically, why has our society gotten it so wrong? And that's what the story of *Whole* is all about. And I'm trying to argue the case that it's not just about what a lot of people think it is—it's not just about money. Money is a major factor—what "sells" generally is the kind of information the public gets. But it's not that simple, and it's not really a conspiracy on the part of institutions. What I have come to believe is that it is really about the way that we understand science, or in fact the way we misunderstand science.

It's a very different way of thinking about what nutrition really means—and what the practice of medicine really means. I'm convinced that if this were known and people really did practice it—and an increasing number of people are now beginning to do that—if that were known we would be able to save a huge fraction of our health-care cost bill. There's nothing like it.

V for Veg: When you mention "conspiracy," how does that dovetail with, say, recent controversies about the Academy of Nutritional Dietetics (formerly ADA) and its corporate sponsorships?

T. Colin Campbell: That organization has shot themselves in the foot—I don't think we can rely on the information they now provide. What they have done is partner with the people that have been putting out so much junk information for so long. When you have Coca-Cola, Pepsi-Cola, GlaxoSmithKline and the dairy industry, when you have those huge big organizations partnering with this so-called professional society, I don't see how anybody can expect to get good information out of that. They window-dress their information to make it look reasonably correct sometimes, but in reality they don't show how nutrition can improve people's health. I've spoken to that group as a keynoter three times over the years. The last time was in 2008, and by the time I got there then, I think the organization had gone over the top.

Now, this may sound like a conflict with what I said previously, that I don't believe in conspiracies, but . . . 'conspiracy' is a case, in my view, where people actually sit around a table, if you will, and concoct up a story and arrange for their trade in defiance of what they really know . . . I don't want to detract from the individual dietitians. They did spend four or five years getting their degrees. They do spend a lot of time learning a lot of information, and I find dietitians to be wonderful people, full of a lot of energy oftentimes and very sincere. But when they're operating within a system that is controlling what they can do and what they can say and what they can practice . . . you see? So I'm speaking out for dietitians and speaking against the institutions that control their training and their practices. I want to be very careful to make that distinction.

Of course, it's not just that institution that I find such fault in—it's basically the way that even larger institutions—you know, government-run institutions and agencies in addition to medical institutions—get caught in this whirlwind of information that's become almost like a tornado, and we're all spinning around with all this information that quite frankly is doing a lot of damage. We've got to step out of that box and think of another way of understanding: What does this really say, what is the evidence, how can we interpret it, how do we design studies, what kind of policies do we make on the basis of the evidence we get? There's so much in this information that we can talk about and actually deliver to the American public so they can actually get well. That's my interest.

V for Veg: Other than your books, are other channels emerging where people will have this info delivered to them?

T. Colin Campbell: Well, I do have a non-profit foundation and we partner with the online program of Cornell University, which is one of the top ten in the country, and we offer what we find to be a very exciting online course in plant-based nutrition. We've been authorized to give 30 class-one credits to doctors, and so about a third of our students now online are physicians and primary health-care workers, so that's one way. And we're finding that to be an exciting kind of thing—and that may sound kind of self-serving but I don't get paid on that, this is just a non-profit thing that we brought some really good people together to do.

As far as other organizations are concerned, there are some potentially very good organizations that could pick up the ball and run in this new direction, but the problem is that as yet they're still too encumbered with corporate influence to break free of those chains. A lot of people would not mind, as with the dieticians [needing an accrediting institution], they would like to have something to hang their hat on before they go out and get too serious about what they're talking about. So I'm just hoping this book, *Whole,* will start a discussion.

Jan 26, 2012

Pssst, Deen Foes: "Vegan" and "Healthy" Are Not Synonyms

When Paula Deen announced her type 2 diabetes last week, outrage erupted worldwide. Coming as healthful New Year's resolutions are eroding like melting snow, the news struck a chord.

That's because Deen had long preached a comfort-food gospel heavy on butter, sugar, meat and other "down-home" delights that many work to minimize.

And she knew her condition for three years before revealing it—once she had a gig hawking diabetes drug Victoza.

As the *New York Times*'s Frank Bruni put it, "She had waited three long, greasy years since her diagnosis to come out. During that period, she promoted the deep-fried life without acknowledging her firsthand experience of how a person can be burned by it."

Food Politics (University of California Press) author Marion Nestle slammed Deen for striking a "common folk" pose while shilling a $500-a-month drug. Even the *Wall Street Journal* weighed in, teasing apart the contradictions of Deen's position from a brand perspective in "Paula Deen Pitch Hard to Swallow."

An unrepentant Deen said she'd given up sweet tea and claimed to have always seasoned her outrageous concoctions (fried butter balls, doughnut-based cheeseburgers, etc.) with a reminder to "practice moderation, y'all."

In the *Albany Times-Union,* Susan Levin shot back: "It's not the sweet tea. It's the butter, the beef and the bacon.... It's time to admit that modest reforms to profoundly unhealthy eating habits will not rescue anyone from diabetes and obesity—even if you throw in a heaping helping of expensive pharmaceuticals."

Deen tried to have it both ways. And ironically, that's what many of my veggie colleagues have been doing.

How? By insisting that Deen should fight her diabetes by "going vegan."

Many claimed such a step would vastly improve Deen's (and her fans') health, if not outright reverse her condition.

But vegan is not synonymous with healthy. And when we imply it is, we're double-dipping, too.

Yes, vegans can have comforting cake, candy and ice cream—and potato chips, french fries, hot dogs and toaster waffles—without sacrifice. And yes, a low-fat, plant-based diet is a key component in dramatically reversing some health conditions.

But realistically, those are two poles: The more rich "comfort" food you eat, the less health benefit you get.

Granted, though, going animal-free ditches dietary cholesterol, cuts saturated fat (less prevalent in plant foods) and ups fiber intake (animal foods have no fiber), so there is a health plus.

And a guiding ethical principle can strengthen the willpower it takes to stick with an eating plan.

Prove it? OK. This year I've made a resolution everyone can share: While easing a tiny bit on vegan treats, I plan to double my consumption of fresh fruits and vegetables. Who's with me?

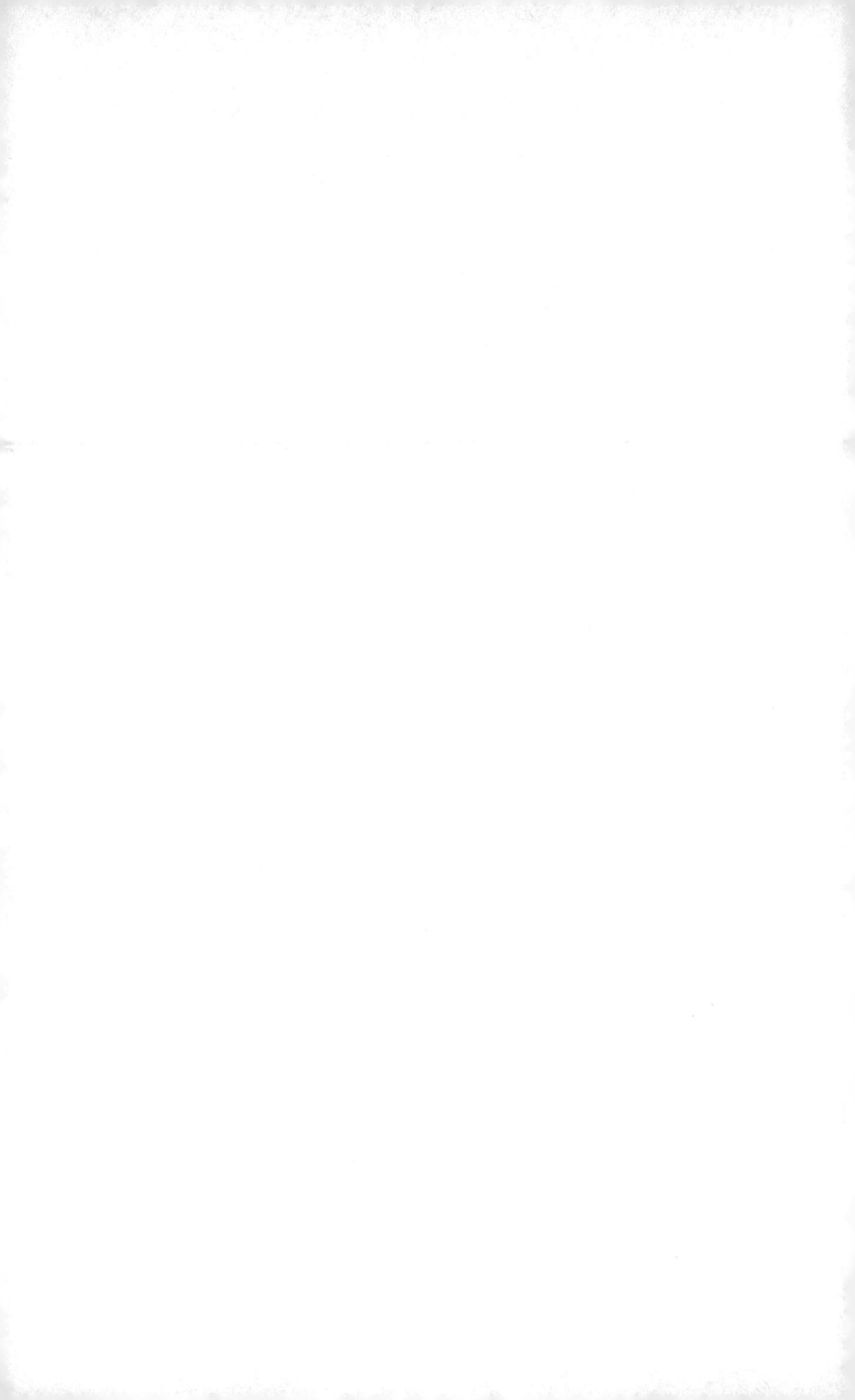

FOOD FAVES

Nov 17, 2011
Vegan Thanksgiving: From Tofurky to the Three Sisters

Free Thanksgiving turkeys!

Who wouldn't agree to that, right?

Unfortunately, freeing Thanksgiving turkeys is both difficult and illegal—but you can "free" the one on your table this year with a turkey-free dinner.

I know, turkey-free Thanksgiving is sacrilege to some, but others are snapping up the new products being introduced to fill a compassionate holiday platter.

Of these, Turtle Island Foods's Tofurky has been around for decades—long enough that the misnomer "tofurkey" is often used for any meatless turkey substitute. The company continually tweaks the overall "Feast" package, which this year includes a delicious Amy's chocolate cake.

Tofurky strikes a balance—serving as a turkey-like centerpiece without trying to imitate one. The uncooked item looks like a formless bag of protein but, as with meat, it's how you prepare it that counts. I not only add the recommended potatoes, carrots and onions to "roast" (bake inside foil) with it, but mix and apply a signature marinade that boosts the overall garlic quotient by about 600 percent and that also makes creditable use of Yuengling Premium.

Shopping tip: Any time you want a Tofurky Feast, go to ShopRite, which stocks them year-round. My local Whole Foods had none out yet when I needed one for this column.

But it did a week later, when it also had Gardein's new T-Day product, Turk'y. These come two to a bag and are self-contained single servings with gravy topping. Each was crispy, hearty and flavorful, but the per-person approach fails as a big holiday centerpiece.

That's exactly where the Vegan Whole Turkey from VegeUSA (www.vegeusa.com) excels. This is a nearly turkey-size soy concoction that looks unnervingly like an actual roasted turkey. One wonders about the appeal: A turkey shape won't draw vegetarians, and no meat-eater is going to be fooled into thinking it's an actual turkey. So as far as that goes, it's just kind of bizarre.

However, with some rudimentary preparation (it comes with gravy and with stuffing that you prepare and then, yes, stuff into the turkey-like thing) this turned out to be very tasty and satisfying: A little more bready than Tofurky but flavorful—and with a flavor not too far from turkey.

Then again, you can have an intensively prepared centerpiece that completely ignores turkey.

Lasagna is a popular Thanksgiving choice for many veggie types. Our family has gone this route a couple of times, and the best lasagna recipe I've found is in Imar Hutchins and Dawn Marie Daniels's *Vegetarian Soul Food Cookbook*.

Imar is right about the key being the fresh-made sauce, but make sure you buy lasagna noodles, an ingredient he forgets to list.

Of all the non-turkey options, Neal Barnard, president of the Physicians' Committee for Responsible Medicine, may have the most appropriate meal plan of all: the "three sisters."

For those who know their early American culinary history (Barnard admits his embarrassment at encountering this only a couple of years ago), the "three sisters" known to various American Indian tribes are corn, beans and squash. Planted together, they grow symbiotically, supporting each other in their diversity. Barnard sees this as a more relevant and meaningful metaphor for gathering one's family to give thanks than is the traditional big-dead-animal centerpiece.

"It's always seemed peculiar, this idea of giving thanks by being a glutton," he said, noting that there are many possible dishes (some may already be on your menu) based on one or more of these three. To name just a few: bean tacos, squash soup, polenta, baked beans, roasted butternut squash, three-bean salad, corn bread, green beans and pumpkin pie. (Though I might opt for the tofu-based chocolate silk pie—hey, soy is a bean!)

Although turkey loyalists constantly invoke "tradition," Barnard said that "it's useful to remember real traditional foods. The Native Americans turned out a pretty good banquet themselves." There are more tips, including a recipe for Smashing Corn Casserole, whose ingredients include the three sisters, at www.pcrm.org.

And to anyone and everyone involved, whether you free a turkey or not, let me be sure to say: Thanks!

Apr 17, 2014
Keeping the Soul, Losing the Meat

Bryant Terry pretty much wrote the book on vegan soul-food cooking, by which I mean 2009's *Vegan Soul Kitchen* (Da Capo). Not that there were no well-done guides to vegan soul food out there, but Terry's had a huge impact in mainstream and vegan worlds—and on Takia McClendon.

About the book the *New York Times* said "makes Southern cooking healthy and cool," McClendon related in a phone interview that "it was my first cookbook as a vegan!" Terry, she said, is "someone who really taught me how to cook," inspiring her efforts to connect her community with soul food that tastes great but omits the health, environmental and ethical downsides of traditional fare.

So when Terry reached out with an idea to collaborate on a Philadelphia book-signing, McClendon was eager to make it work.

He's coming here to promote the new *Afro-Vegan: Farm-Fresh African, Caribbean, and Southern Flavors Remixed* (Ten Speed Press), and the event, hosted by McClendon's Uptown Soul Food, will be a sit-down dinner at Germantown's Soup Factory Studio.

McClendon launched Uptown Soul Food in 2011 with a mission "to serve fresh, creative, plant-based cuisine while celebrating and upholding traditional African-American culinary history."

In addition to meal-planning and catering, an Uptown series of "pop-up" restaurant events at the now-closed Wired Beans Cafe featured vegan versions of comfort foods such as chicken sandwiches and macaroni and cheese.

At next week's supper, "vegetables are more central to the menu," McClendon said. She laughed when I referenced the upscale restaurant Vedge, and replied that, while no one will confuse this food with Rich Landau's cooking, it is an endeavor "to introduce high-quality, plant-based food" to people who are not going to Vedge or HipCityVeg. "All the dishes will be from *Afro-Vegan*, such as a mustard-greens salad with an oil-free vinaigrette.

"Mustard greens are often used in soul food," McClendon said, "but African-Americans tend to cook 'em to death."

Here, the bitter tang of the greens is balanced by strong flavors of garlic, yellow onion, tomato paste and hot-pepper vinegar, so that while "the greens are a key ingredient, they wind up taking more of a background role."

This kind of reinvention of soul-food cuisine is Terry's signature. His creations appeal because he's remixing "flavors and spices traditionally associated with African-American cooking" rather than simply swapping in "a chick'n burger from Gardein or something," McClendon said.

She has other supper clubs in mind for later in the year, bringing in local chefs to "cook plant-based versions of their favorite dishes," and Uptown Soul Food will be expanding its cooking classes and food demonstrations around Germantown. For now, though, she's concentrating on creating a fantastic event next Monday with Terry.

It's a logical collaboration: Terry's creations tie together distinct cuisines from the African diaspora, "tracing their history and giving them cultural context," as his bio notes, and "building community around the food we prepare and eat."

Bringing together people from around Germantown (and foodies from around Philadelphia) to bond on issues of food justice, healthy eating and all-around deliciousness, McClendon is doing likewise.

Nov 6, 2014
Putting the "Fun" in Fungi
'Shrooms Are Plentiful, Beautiful... Go Forage, but Watch What You Eat

On a recent Saturday afternoon, I finally went hunting.

I was outfitted to fight the elements and loaded for—not bear, but certainly hen of the woods and other kinds of wild-growing edible mushrooms.

Armed with a knife and an old grocery bag, I set out with fungi enthusiast and local photographer Michele Frentrop and expert mushroom collector Felix Giordano to earn our food just like our ancestors did.

Well, Felix's ancestors, anyway. I doubt mine ever had a plant-based meal that didn't originate in a freezer.

It was a cool, misty day, which Frentrop said was good, both as a mood-setter and because "we can see the mushrooms better without sunshine."

There'd be less foraging competition, too, she added.

Oh, right. I should mention two things here:

Where we were headed for was "somewhere in the Pine Barrens"—you'll get nothing more specific than that out of me. Forager's code, man.

And, of course, do not read this story and head out on your own looking for edible mushrooms. You must have a Felix Giordano or local equivalent with you. He, by the way, has been collecting mushrooms in the Pine Barrens since he was six. Now 68, he was schooled by his dad and uncle.

A quick review: There are poisonous mushrooms and nonpoisonous ones. It takes an expert eye to tell them apart.

Within that second category are "edible" and "inedible" varieties. The latter won't hurt you but are either too tough for eating or just flavorless. Some people also have allergic reactions to one mushroom type or another, Giordano noted.

Most authorities agree that all mushrooms should be cooked before eating. "There are only two kinds I would eat raw," said Giordano. "White button mushrooms and chicken [of-the-woods, a different variety than hen], if it was really fresh."

This was relevant because we had ventured only a few feet into the pines when we found some chicken-of-the-woods that was, unfortunately, too old to bother with, its taste and chewability having reached shoe-leather levels.

When fresh, the bright, tannish-orange chicken "looks like chicken cutlets," Giordano said. It can be used in place of chicken in some dishes.

Further ahead, I found an interesting cluster of golden-brown mushrooms on a rotting log. But when I pointed them out to Giordano, he just shrugged.

"Yeah. LBMs." Little Brown Mushrooms.

These, I learned, are all the varieties you don't care about identifying because they're most likely either poisonous or inedible. Fascinating to a professional mycologist, perhaps; they're junk finds for our expert forager, because if you don't wanna eat 'em, what's the point?

"I know about 10 to 12 different kinds of mushrooms really well that grow around here," Giordano explained, offhandedly. "The others I just don't bother with."

He pointed out a couple of chubby, slimy slippery jacks (*Suillus luteus*), barely discernible beneath some dead leaves. "Those are OK for eating," he said.

He then saw a couple of attractive white mushrooms standing tall out of the leaves like fully opened umbrellas. "Those are some kind of amanitas," he said, with a shrug. It wasn't worth trying to identify them further because they would either be bad-tasting or outright poisonous.

The slippery jacks were plentiful, much more so than the honey mushrooms (*Armillaria mellea*) that Frentrop and Giordano had thought would be out. (They did go back the next weekend and found "a lot of honeys," they later told me.)

"My folks used to call [the jacks] porcini," mused Giordano. "They're in the boletus family." He explained that mushrooms tend to pick up different common names in different places. Hen-of-the-woods (*Grifola frondosa*) is known in Japan as maitake.

More than once, Frentrop hoisted a specimen to my nose and asked me to smell. "Earthy, isn't it?" she enthused. I had to agree: yeah, earthy, got it.

By midday, our trio was more dispersed throughout the silent, misty pine forest, though within seeing/hearing distance, and still not more than a few yards from the road. I was now more confident in looking on my own, though I still wouldn't touch anything without corroboration.

At one point, I checked the back side of a rotting stump and found a cluster of mushrooms sporting light-brown caps with a distinctive, reddish-brown coloring in the middle. I called to Giordano, who quickly and enthusiastically identified them as brick tops (*Hypholoma sublateritium*).

"Good eating," he added.

Frentrop and I saw a couple of *Amanita muscaria* (fly agaric), which are so freakishly colorful—reddish-orange tops with whitish polka dots—that they look like the classic cartoon toadstool.

"Some places it's called the stupefying mushroom," Giordano said, because of its hallucinogenic effect. "You can make a bug spray out of it. It won't kill the bug, it will just get them stoned."

We continued gathering slippery jacks into the late afternoon. By now, it was easy for me to spot them hiding in the leaves.

We wound up with enough mushrooms to fill a milk crate, divvied them up and headed home. Frentrop helped me cook the slippery jacks in oil, thyme and wine. I also sautéed the brick tops in garlic.

We put the mushrooms in pitas and took a bite.

Maybe it was the long, long day, the hours of walking. Maybe it was the misty forest. Maybe it was the satisfaction of having caught our own food. But that was the best-tasting mushroom sandwich I've ever had.

Texture-wise it was less award-winning: The slippery jacks stayed slippery, since we had been too exhausted to peel the slimy top off each cap before cooking. Frentrop offered that a better use for these would be in a sauce or soup.

Still, I was satisfied, especially as I reflected on a day spent connecting with autumn in all its slow-changing glory—orange, brown, red and yellow hues splashed across a multitude of different organisms, some dying, others thriving on their passage.

Somehow mushrooms, with their earthy quality, seem to bring all that to your plate.

May 31, 2012
Vegan Boy Meets Grill

You know veganism has arrived when even newspaper comic-strip characters are taking the plunge. Last week in the Philly-set "Jump Start," Sunny, the precocious family daughter, proclaimed her intent to veganize, citing her aunt Charlene as already vegan.

But it's also no surprise that both characters are female: To many people, vegan equals "girly," a notion borne out by a recent marketing study that found both men and women often ascribe manliness to meat and daintiness to tofu ("Is Meat Male? A Quantitative Multi-Method Framework to Establish Metaphoric Relationships," *Journal of Consumer Research,* October 2012).

It's an age-old prejudice Carol Adams so deftly covered in *The Sexual Politics of Meat* (Bloomsbury Academic) more than 20 years ago.

But a new cookbook from John Schlimm, *Grilling Vegan Style* (Da Capo), throws stereotypes into the flames, fusing that icon of he-man tech, the outdoor grill, with meat-free foods—all slathered with Schlimm's signature saucy style.

"Yes, it is cliché how 'grill' and 'macho' are synonymous in some people's minds," Schlimm said in an email interview, "much like 'grill' and 'meat' have always been synonymous . . . until now!"

This hard-partying author (remember last year's *The Tipsy Vegan,* also from Da Capo?) always manages to sound like he's leaning into your face and elbowing you in the ribs, though with good-natured zest: "Consider *Grilling Vegan Style* my SIZZLING dissertation on how the grill is now a place where barriers are torn down, whether we're talking about gender / who is serving as grill master, or food / what fantastic plant-based ingredients are being tossed on the flames."

His new book covers the basics of grilling (with a comprehensive guide to grills) and is stocked with animal-free burger and kebab recipes. (Try one at Philly.com/grillvegan.) It also encourages readers to be adventurous and grill just about everything—apples, peaches, salads, watermelons and even peanut-butter-and-jelly sandwiches.

If a male reader wants to be "manly" about it, Schlimm points to chapters 8 ("The Burgers Are Ready!") and 9 ("The New Tailgating Classics"). But, he added, "I would warn them, women will ROCK those recipes and chapters just as well!"

Schlimm's philosophy "is that this is a party EVERYONE is invited to: vegans and carnivores, men and women, young and old, backyard dwellers and beach bums—the only requirement is that you have to want to have FUN."

Of course, Schlimm and his cruelty-free grill aren't alone: The reality of "manly" vegan men is running roughshod over the clichés, with guys like hunky Texas firefighter/vegan advocate Rip Esselstyn on the front lines, and a posse of vegan jocks redefining "tough" as boxers, bodybuilders, ultramarathoners and Ironman triathletes.

A recent study ("Carotenoid and melanin pigment coloration affect perceived human health," *Evolution and Human Behaviour,* 2010) found women preferring men's faces that had a "healthy" look (skin glowing from what the researchers cite as a diet high in fruits and vegetables) over those that looked "macho."

And once a guy gets with his chosen partner . . . again, the documented reality of meat-eating shows the popular fantasy to be somewhat flaccid.

Victoria Moran's new book, *Main Street Vegan* (TarcherPerigee), puts it succinctly: "Meat is connected to virility, but it's negatively connected. The more meat—and cheese, and eggs and fried foods—a guy eats, the less likely he is to enjoy a full and satisfying sex life for as long as he wants one."

So fellas, are you brave, strong and confident? Prove it by conquering the primordial fear of tofu on the grill.

Aug 7, 2014
Still Time to Rake in Your Own Fresh Veggies

Everyone agrees on the value of fresh fruits and vegetables, especially locally sourced, and this is the time of year when farmers markets overflow with green beans, corn, tomatoes, blackberries and blueberries. Fully embracing the source of your food is natural for vegans. When not patronizing local farms, many of us grow our own.

For instance, in my own garden this year . . .

Omigod, that's right! I was so busy pontifica—er, educating—that I didn't get around to planting anything this spring. There's nothing in our three 6-by-6 raised beds but weeds!

Oh man, is it too late?

I threw this question out to everyone I knew, including my lovely wife, Cynthia, who reminded me that we can still plant my favorite leafy green, kale, well into September. I took to Twitter and got a bushel of other suggestions—broccoli, cabbage, lettuce, herbs, radishes...

Radishes. I used to love them as a kid but I never seem to get them at the store these days. So, they're the perfect food to grow: Even if one can't live on radishes alone, they have proven benefits, such as enabling rude boys to burp most of the alphabet.

I persuaded Cynthia to help me get the garden back in shape for a late planting. In just a few weeks we can be feasting on radishes. And after that, kale.

The first thing we found: two "volunteers," dill and tomato, coming up in spite of our slackery. So, we've already got a head start on, well, some kind of tomato-dill salad. We worked around those and turned up the earth elsewhere. I just wanted to clear a couple of rows for radishes. Cynthia had acquired seeds for those, plus Swiss chard, spinach, fennel, cabbage, arugula, collards, parsley, mustard, Brussels sprouts, rutabaga and bok choy.

As for my favorite, "They were out of kale," she reported.

I muttered, "Damn hipsters."

Now she had me raking the dirt to level the growing field. "You don't want big clods on the surface," she noted. I remembered how, our first year, a footprint of about my shoe size remained in the middle of the bed through the growing season from one errant step back in the planting phase. Big clods, indeed.

Next task was to dig out some compost and mix with wet potting soil. Our compost pile is somewhat haphazard. I came across shreds of a potato-chip bag—who the heck put that in there?—then I realized it was the infamous ultra-loud Sun Chips bag from 2010 that assaulted eardrums across America but was "100% compostable"! So far it was still vibrant colored and mostly intact, not something I wanted to add to the garden. I'll admit, though, that its crackle was no longer so loud.

Cynthia reminded me to place a little stick next to where each seedling would come up—right after I had gotten them all put in. I guesstimated. She chuckled and shook her head, then wound up doing the same thing. It's a tricky process.

One downside of starting plants in August is that the average rainfall is less than, say, in March, April or May, so be ready to keep the dirt moist (on sunny days, morning and/or evening, never midday). We lucked out in that it started raining as soon as we got everything in.

Looking out over the smooth soil beds filled with various potential after a hard day's work, we cracked a couple of cold ones and relished the coming bounty.

The point, I realized, is to not give up, even when you think it might be too late.

May 17, 2012
Get Fruit and Veggies the Easy Way: Drinking

How're those New Year's resolutions going? Back in January, I challenged myself, and you, to double our fruit and vegetable intake by the end of 2012. And as of this month, I pretty much already have.

OK, partly that's because my total for fresh fruit has historically been pitiful. But I also had a powerful ally that gave me confidence: a Vitamix high-speed blender.

In just a few months, I've had so many fruit and vegetable smoothies that I've already passed my 2011 total.

Have these healthful drinks turned me slim and fit and trim? Uh, we'll get to that.

But first, it's not exactly breaking news that smoothies have been gaining in popularity and market share. You can get one on practically any corner in Center City. Starbucks and McDonald's sell them. But I knew smoothies had truly arrived with the publication a couple of weeks ago of *The Complete Idiot's Guide to Green Smoothies* (Alpha).

This book by Bo Rinaldi evangelizes for the health-promoting power of green smoothies but never goes over the top, sticking to sound nutrition science. Smoothies, he notes, are a great way to get a smorgasbord of phytonutrients in an easily digestible form that tastes great. As long as, you know, you make sure it tastes great. To that end, the book is stocked with 150 recipes ranging from the everyday to the exotic, all with front-loaded info on key nutrients per smoothie.

Two caveats: While the mantra is that smoothies are quick and easy, set aside time to get the process down. The prep, mixing and cleanup may take some time before you find your groove. And then there's the lack of chewing.

In January, the Happy Herbivore blog touched off a mini-tempest by citing Caldwell Esselstyn (the *Forks Over Knives* doctor) dissing smoothies compared with eating whole fruits and vegetables. Chewing, you see, stimulates our digestive enzymes; not chewing allows plant sugars to go straight into our system, potentially causing a spike in glucose. There also may be some loss of effectiveness in finely pureed fiber.

But as Rinaldi points out, you can mitigate the first by "pretend[ing] to chew for just a moment" as you start sipping "to ensure the most complete digestion." As for getting the fiber and vitamins in a smoothie, in my case that needs to be compared, realistically, with not getting them at all. For me and probably many others, the benefits we get from smoothies do not replace whole, intact foods, but rather, replace zilch.

The archetypal green smoothie may be the blend of kale and apple—one for diverse nutrients (kale packs legendary vitamin power, though its cousin spinach is also very potent and popular), the other for a tart sweetness to round off the leaf's bitter edge. These two alone are enough to make a basic smoothie.

From there you might lean more in a vegetable (i.e., savory) direction by adding parsley, spinach, tomato, onion, garlic and cucumber, or you might head more for the sweet fruit effect with frozen strawberries, raspberries, blueberries, mango, cantaloupe and banana. In general, you get a better bang for the calories with vegetables, because fruits, while also nutrient-rich, also tend to be sugar-rich.

Again, I don't eat a lot of doughnuts, so if I can get fruits in a tasty though caloric form, for me that's a net gain. Your mileage might vary. For now my best signature smoothie is fruit-based—bananas, strawberries and blueberries with just a hint of kale. You'd be surprised what you can add kale and spinach to for an extra vitamin kick.

Although Vitamix is the well-loved pioneer in home high-speed blenders, there's also Blendtec, which I haven't tried but has its own fervent partisans. You can use an ordinary, lower-speed blender, but Rinaldi cautions that you should layer ingredients more carefully so you don't burn out the motor.

If there's one argument for springing for a high-speed blender, it's ice cream. A handful of pecans and almonds, some agave nectar, vanilla and spice combine with a tray of ice cubes to create an out-of-this-world dessert treat in about 30 seconds. Technically it's a sorbet (no dairy products), but your tongue will scream "ice cream!" That's because the fat in the nuts has been pulverized along with the ice crystals to generate a smoothness not far from butterfat.

Once I mastered this simple, scrumptious concoction, all hope of Vitamix-based weight-loss was also pulverized.

But don't worry: Little by little, I'm going to start adding kale to it!

Jan 10, 2013
Rock the Crock
Meatless Dishes, Even Pizza, from a Slow Cooker

When it's cold outside, there's nothing like coming home to the warming aroma of a slow-cooked meal, a simmering mixture subtly blending the flavors and colors of potatoes, carrots, beans, rice, squash, tomatoes, corn, mushrooms, onions, spices . . .

But wait, where's the meat?

A fair question: After all, just about everybody who was around in the 1970s recalls that tenderizing and flavor-boosting cheap cuts of meat was a main selling point in slow cookers' original launch and rise. Less well-known is the fact that the appliance churning out those pot roasts, beef stews and chicken cacciatores was originally conceived as a bean cooker.

In the mid-'60s, modeling West Bend's somewhat similar Bean Pot, Naxon Utilities Corp. introduced a slow cooker pitched for baked beans and chili, called the Beanery. Rival purchased Naxon in 1970 and a year later reintroduced the Beanery with a new name: Crock-Pot. Now emphasizing tenderized-meat recipes, the new appliance soon became the go-to option for one-pot meals assembled in the morning and enjoyed in the evening, especially as the rise of double-income households meant less time for supper preparations.

Its simple low/medium/high controls, general ease of use and groovy color schemes made the Crock-Pot ubiquitous in American kitchens for a while. The "fad" aspect wore off long ago, but slow cookers continue to sell.

The slow cooker's endurance is due in part to continuing improvements, such as built-in timers and a lower "keep warm" setting, that expanded the appliance's flexibility. But its attraction also lies in its ability to prepare a wide variety of vegetarian and vegan meals more easily and healthfully (very little oil is needed, for instance) than most other methods.

Two recent cookbooks attest to this: *Quick and Easy Vegan Slow Cooking: More than 150 Tasty, Nourishing Recipes That Practically Make Themselves* by Carla Kelly (The Experiment) and Robin Robertson's *Fresh from the Vegan Slow Cooker: 200 Ultra-Convenient, Super-Tasty, Completely Animal-Free Recipes* (Harvard Common Press).

If you think of this cuisine as just removing the meat from an existing dish, leaving a bunch of bland, mushy vegetables, you're missing out.

First, that "bland mush" danger is yours to minimize. "Don't overcook!" advised Allyson Kramer, a popular gluten-free-food blogger in Philly who did a slow-cooker series in October. That's especially true with starchy foods like potatoes or lentils. Kramer noted that "many people have preconceived notions about slow cookers," especially when it comes to vegetable-based dishes.

The amount of liquid used also is a factor, since it doesn't evaporate away. Also, familiarizing yourself with the particulars of your unit's cooking time will yield better results.

Stews, chili, soups, curries, dal, goulash—these all fit under the "mushy" rubric, and slow cookers handle them with ease. But Robertson and Kelly show how you can also make spiced nuts, stuffing, risotto, polenta, lasagna, meatless loaf, soy sausage, seitan ribs, lentil pate, pudding, granola, quiche, chocolate peanut-butter cheesecake and pizza.

That's right, pizza.

OK, you can't fit a cookie sheet in a slow cooker, so we're not talking the thin, crispy-crust variety, but you can make an extra-large personal-pan pizza such as Robertson's deep-dish olives-and-capers Pizza Puttanesca.

Robertson's book abounds with newly adapted recipes to expand your slow-cooker repertoire, as well as good advice on the pros and cons of this technology: "Hard vegetables, such as onions and carrots, added raw to soups will soften well because of the amount of liquid they are cooking in. However, if those same vegetables are added raw to a stew-type dish, they may remain hard long after the rest of the ingredients are cooked because there is not as much liquid for them to cook in."

Robertson often recommends giving harder veggies "a head start by sautéing them first for a few minutes in a little water or oil to soften them a bit."

Another tip for uniform cooking is to cut harder ingredients into smaller pieces, she said. "The smaller or thinner you cut or slice ingredients, the more quickly they will cook."

Conversely, adding certain elements near the end (e.g. fresh greens or herbs, and sometimes rice and pasta) creates textural contrast and flavor depth. And, once you become familiar with timing issues like these, you can get even more out of your device.

Perhaps the most surprising thing about a slow cooker, Robertson noted, is that it can be used to make desserts. "Sure, you might expect that it makes great bread pudding or even baked apples," she said. "But you can also use it to make cobblers, cakes and even cheesecakes—all without turning on the oven. I like to see the expressions of people when I tell them the cheesecake they're enjoying not only contains no dairy, but was also 'baked' in a slow cooker."

Granted, the more creative you get with a slow cooker, the further you're getting from the "set it and forget it" ethos. But many of these excursions fit into the category of 20-minute prep in the morning plus a bit more when you get home—still a big difference from starting dinner from scratch at that point.

As Kelly notes in her book intro, the "quick and easy" part comes at "the end of the day, when you have less energy and really can't face the idea of cooking."

Slow cooking is a rewarding and forgiving method that gives good results for beginners, and it can be tweaked, with experience, to excellent effect. As Kramer put it, "Quality ingredients, herbs and spices chosen appropriately, proper vegetable preparation and a little know-how are all you need to create a wonderful meal."

5 Quick Crock Tips

1. Slow cookers vary in size, and every unit has a small variability in cooking times. Allow extra cooking time while you learn the particulars of your device.
2. A Crock-Pot's ceramic insert is hardy, but it can crack. Always thaw frozen food before adding to the pot. And allow the insert to cool before washing, especially if you're using cold water.
3. Kidney beans should be brought to a boil before slow cooking to destroy a toxin that low-temperature cooking won't. The toxin, with the unpronounceable name of phytohaemagglutinin, causes digestive distress. Easier, of course, is to use canned, precooked kidney beans.
4. Some vegetables will retain more vitamins if they are blanched or sautéed briefly before being added to the mix.

5. Tofu tends to fall apart in most slow-cooker recipes unless added near the end; conversely, tempeh holds up well and tends to become less bitter and more flavorful in a slow-cooked environment.

Nov 29, 2012

Recipe Remakes for Vegan Junk-Food Junkies

If you started November as a junk-food junkie, it was kind of a rough month.

Papa John's threatened a 14-cent-per-pizza hike. A Denny's franchise (soon contradicted by the parent company) promised a similar 5 percent surcharge. And Hostess, in a fight over union benefits, pulled the plug entirely. All just after President Obama's re-election.

Geez, does First Lady Michelle Obama's healthier-foods crusade really wield so much clout?

If only. Whether economic outcry or post-election posturing, these blips won't budge the monolith of U.S. junk food. But they remind us that the "traditional America"—cheap standard-issue pizza and snack treats dominating our nation's plates and minds—may not last forever.

Already pizza is diversifying, with vegan and gluten-free options showing up in regular pizza shops. These pizzas may not be "health food," but you can actually find those in *Heart Healthy Pizza* by Mark Sutton (CreateSpace Independent Publishing Platform).

Sutton finds ways to replicate pizza's zesty charm without added oils or fats, a key to optimal heart health. He explains how to build cheesy sauces from bases such as barley, black-eyed peas, tofu, potatoes or almonds.

So maybe pizza can actually be a good-for-you food. But what about stuff like Twinkies?

We know the Twinkie will live on somewhere, somehow, as someone else makes their version. But if it's an ersatz "Twinkie," why not make your own?

Renowned pastry chef Fran Costigan was demonstrating just that back in 2007 on network TV. In a fun "Nightline" segment on ABC (5/3/2007), Costigan deftly showed that eggs and dairy, which are pumped into such dessert treats (along with beef fat[!] in Twinkies) are not necessary to make a great-tasting sweet spongy dessert.

I was clued into this by Sharon Nazarian's blog Big City Vegan (Philly.com/bcvegan), and chatted with Costigan recently when she was in town—our own Running Press will be publishing her 2013 cookbook devoted to chocolate.

Costigan is no fan of low-fat desserts. "What's the point?" she said. "If you cut out the fat, you have to use four or five times as much sugar." Instead she swaps elements here and there, using "healthier alternatives" that don't interfere with the basic taste and feel.

I've sampled Costigan's wares and can attest to her wizardry in maintaining flavor, sweetness and texture while cutting out the worst elements of the originals. So if she could tweak the Twinkie... could she fake a Tastykake?

Yes! Check out Costigan's KandyKakes variations. She warns that hers, which use organic ingredients without chemical stabilizers, won't taste exactly the same—"They taste better."

If you want to tip more into the "junky" realm, you might like Lane Gold's *Vegan Junk Food* from Adams Media, which touts "sinful snacks that are good for the soul," including dairy-free Boston Cream Pie and vegan Philly cheesesteaks.

With a little effort, you can cut both the animals and the millionaire junk-food CEOs out of the equation, creating your own healthier, delicious—and surprisingly affordable—"junk" food.

Or you can just swing by Blackbird Pizzeria and snag some Vegan Treats.

It takes all kinds, right?

Nov 20, 2014
No Harm, No Fowl
Out of Many Dishes, a New Unity

Back in the Norman Rockwell days, Thanksgiving dinner was unified. All eyes at the table hungrily focused on that giant roast turkey that Grandma was placing on the table, everybody with a single thought:

Gimme.

Nowadays, there's your gluten-free cousin, your soy-allergic aunt, somebody's lactose-intolerant boyfriend, a niece who shuns meat for ethical reasons.

Unity is gone—how can you make one meal to satisfy all these requirements?

Now imagine you're trying to satisfy not a handful but 300 people. That was the task for Rachel Klein, whose plant-based creative chops at Philly's Miss Rachel's Pantry won her the prestige gig of Thanksliving 2014, a renowned celebration at the Woodstock Farm Animal Sanctuary, in Woodstock, NY.

Klein created the main-course menu and ran the kitchen to bring the dishes to life on Thanksliving Day, October 12.

The Woodstock dinner is a festive reunion for vegans across the Northeast (along with their nonvegan friends!) and a fundraiser for the sanctuary, which houses rescued farm animals and celebrated its 10th anniversary this year.

Overseen by WFAS founders Jenny Brown and Doug Abel, Thanksliving is held in a giant tent in the middle of a goat field and kicks off with a ceremonial turkey dinner—that is, dinner lovingly fed to the handful of resident turkeys on-site.

The Thanksliving menu was 100 percent animal-free, but those in charge know how it is to feel left out at the big table, so they went the extra mile to make it more inclusive. Klein had experience from the Farmhouse Table communal dinners she serves at her Passyunk Avenue restaurant and catering company, and she made substituting friendlier alternatives seem easy.

"For simplicity's sake," Klein told me, "I did the whole thing [tree]nut-free. I'm used to doing that at the restaurant."

What about soy?

"I love using tofu and soy milk and I don't want to vilify soy," she said, but she's found that "it's really kind of easy not to use it."

She made all the Thanksliving dishes without soy, though the main protein, a Pumpkin Seed-Dusted Chickpea-Seitan Roast, did include tamari, which typically contains soybeans and wheat.

For the gluten-sensitive, Klein created a main-dish alternative: tempeh-lentil roast. Her Brussels sprouts salad was also gluten-free.

Lactose is a more common issue than many realize, as the majority of the world's adults are lactose intolerant. Likewise, cow's milk is one of the most common food allergens for kids, so you can feed two birds with one pie by going dairy-free wherever you can.

Klein made a delicious sweet potato bisque that used coconut milk to creamy advantage. "Coconut milk goes nicely with baked potato," Klein observed. "It worked well in the potato bisque. And it was going to be soy milk for the au gratin potatoes, but I wound up using coconut there as well."

Coconut is not a universal solution, as coconut allergies, though relatively rare, do exist. You might want to canvas family members to clear it. Even Klein wound up making a couple of special meals, despite her inclusive main menu.

With the volume and the specialization, Thanksliving was no piece of vegan cake. Klein and her right-hand woman, Carley Leibowitz, worked with about a dozen volunteers in a "giant kitchen" over three days to get everything perfect. The result was a sumptuous, bountiful meal that could not have been improved, diners agreed.

I lucked into sitting with Elissa Katz, one of two Philly women (the other is Marianne Bessey) responsible for Kayli, the cow that got loose in Upper Darby in 2011, getting a home at WFAS. Katz pronounced the meal an unqualified success, whether you knew you were eating soy-free, animal-free, gluten-free, etc.

"It was simply delicious food," she said.

Fran Costigan, the desserts diva behind *Vegan Chocolate* (Running Press), called out the potatoes au gratin in particular as "amazing" and enthused that the "adorable" Klein brings "such a plus to any event, especially this one!"

Klein herself was exhausted by the time I talked to her after dinner, but she had advice for home cooks on the issue of substitutions and inclusiveness at family holiday dinners.

She said it helps to be flexible—maybe a given dish doesn't have to be exactly like grandma made it—and to have "ingredients on hand that you can use in more than one way," such as coconut milk and maple syrup, which can flavor sweet or savory dishes.

Also good at this grateful and helpful holiday is to keep the big picture in mind: Those oddball "problem" eaters aren't veto votes on a scorecard or potholes on the road to culinary perfection, but friends and family—real individuals who got stuck with different constitutions than you. The same, of course, goes for most of WFAS's animal residents.

Which is why making dishes inclusively plant-based is a win-win: More individuals are happy after eating, and more are happy not to be eaten.

Widening our T-Day repertoire to make dishes everyone can enjoy, we can create a new unity, not around a monolithic tradition but around shared values of compassion, justice and awareness.

How does that saying go?

Oh yeah—*E pluribus unum.*

PHILLY-CENTRIC

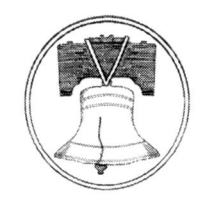

Oct 20, 2011
Ready to Vedge
Owners Broadening Horizons at New Vegan Eatery

If Vedge, the "vegetable restaurant," wasn't Philadelphia's most highly anticipated unveiling when announced, it surely is by now. Despite early promises of a "late summer" debut, it will still be another week before Philadelphians can try this next step from the people behind Horizons.

So what took so long?

"It's excruciating," chef/co-owner Rich Landau admitted last week. "We wanted to be open a month ago, and I can only send out my apology to anyone who's missed a special date or an experience at Horizons or Vedge. We really want to be open for you."

When they started this project, said Kate Jacoby, Landau's partner and wife, "I wish we had asked more questions." There were many logistical and legal issues with the historic building at 1221 Locust, sticking the couple with a major roll of red tape and pushing the projected opening to November 1.

What makes this more than a simple delay is the affection and loyalty many area diners felt toward Horizons, which closed at the beginning of July.

When it opened off South Street in early 2006 (after a decade as Horizons Cafe in Willow Grove), Landau promised "a serious dining adventure" and told me he hoped to establish "Philadelphia's signature vegetarian restaurant." By the time he and Jacoby announced the move to Vedge, Horizons had become all that and more.

Sure, vegans celebrated—*VegNews* (Nov/Dec 2006, #52) named Horizons "Restaurant of the Year" soon after its Philly debut—but the appeal was wider and deeper: *Philadelphia* magazine routinely listed Horizons among its "Top 50 Restaurants," and the *New York Times* ("36 Hours in Philadelphia," 11/26/2006) called it "one of the city's best new restaurants." Landau and Jacoby served the first—and second—all-vegan special-event meals (November 2009, June 2010) at the world-renowned James Beard House in New York City.

So why tinker with perfection?

"Listen, Horizons worked for us," Landau admitted. "People said, 'Oh, you had all these great reviews' [*Inquirer* restaurant critic Craig LaBan, no vegetarian, awarded three bells], and all that . . . but we're not messing with this too much. In fact, people who come here, once they sit down and taste our food, they'll say, 'Well, nothing's really changed.'"

And yet there are changes.

From the two-floor, two-room eatery back at South Street, ground-floor Vedge has evolved into five distinct rooms with different functions. And then there are the plates of food.

Although some early press implied that Vedge would be all greens, leaves and sprouts, that's far from the case. The difference isn't so much in the ingredients as the proportions—and the portions.

Moving away from the "big hunk of protein"-centered entrée, Vedge will feature a greater variety of smaller (and cheaper) dishes that can be combined in twos or threes, tapas-style, for a meal. Although tofu and seitan will not, as some expected, be thrown under the bus, they will "take a back seat," as Landau put it.

"As much as we felt that our big plates really were unique and stood up," he said, "we wanted to make everything more approachable. At Horizons, some people never tried our braciole or our hearts of palm cake because they would always order the grilled seitan or the Pacific Rim tofu." (Guilty as charged!)

"I think a lot of people never wanted to make the commitment to try new things because it was an entrée size—like the last mushroom dish we had: It was a whole roasted maitake mushroom over a stew of fingerling potatoes and leek ash. It was one of my favorite entrées we've ever done, yet a lot of people didn't order it because it is a commitment on a plate.

"Now as a smaller portion, they're going to be able to mix and match and get a lot of different tastes of Vedge."

So if vegetables are coming to the forefront in these dishes, what about desserts? Jacoby explained: "When I first started as pastry chef, I thought the desserts should all be fruit, all fruit. [I thought] people don't want a vegan cheesecake, they want to have, like, a tart—but no, people did want the 'surprise, it's vegan!' cheesecake, crème brûlée, ice cream."

She stepped up to meet that demand, and Horizons's vegan crème brûlée became part of its claim to fame. Given that accomplishment, "we're not going to give up on any of that," she said, but Vedge will have "a little more playful" variety of desserts.

"I think the trick is to put fruit, and maybe some vegetables, into a little bit more of a spotlight with the dessert menu."

Wait a minute—vegetables?

"I've got it," Landau chimed in. "Carrot cake!"

Laughing, Jacoby promised their new, deluxe ice cream maker will be a big part of this equation. "We're going to have some killer ice cream, so that's one way we're going to get playful with our flavors."

The two know playfulness won't be enough to make this move into an unqualified win, especially now that they're moving into the heart of Center City "with the big boys," as Landau put it. There are huge expectations, especially with the extra two months' wait.

"One advantage they have," observed New York's Bart Potenza, "is they're both chefs and cooks. When it's chef-driven, it's easier."

He's talking about the process of opening a new restaurant based on an old one a few blocks away, and he should know: He and partner Joy Pierson have run Candle Cafe, NYC's signature vegan restaurant, since 1994. In 2003 they opened a more upscale version on 79th Street, Candle 79. They're about to release the *Candle 79 Cookbook*.

Potenza and Pierson have been watching the progress from Horizons to Vedge with interest. "I think what they're doing is phenomenal," said Pierson. "They're both so talented, and we love how they represent the mission and the message: veganism, great food, great taste, fresh from farm to table."

Although any restaurant would gladly back a "great food, great taste" mission, veganism continues to be more than a dining category for Landau and Jacoby. As she said, "Rich and I originally got into this for animal-rights reasons." And he pointed out that creating delicious vegan food is their form of low-key activism.

"The message will always be there, underneath, but we're not going to have someone dressed up in a cow suit with a 'Meat is Murder' sign on the sidewalk. You have to lead by example, quietly go about your work and do it well, and people will take notice."

Jacoby noted that they're "demonstrating that [vegan eating] can be this easy," as shown by thousands of surprised and delighted diners who have reconsidered their "need" for animal foods after a meal at Horizons.

So in the end, despite all the hoopla and hand-wringing over delays, despite the razzle-dazzle of a cocktail room and a vegetable bar, it all comes back to the food. And once you decide on your plates, you'll find familiar, delicious flavors.

"It's how I've cooked for 17 years," Landau said. "We're not doing any new techniques, we're not doing molecular gastronomy, we're not going raw or macro. It's going to be Horizons food. We changed just because it's time to change, because you have to change to keep moving and keep growing and keep waking up inspired each day."

*

How Vedge Created Its Signature Dishes
What makes Vedge Vedge and not Horizons? Rich Landau explained the thinking behind three of Vedge's signature dishes:

Little leaves and herbs, rutabaga, smoked shiitake, pistachio, green onion.

"The entry-level dish into the Vedge repertoire, but when you get into it, this is probably one of the more intricate things on the menu because of the way we put it together.

"You won't just be eating a bunch of green. You're not going to taste chlorophyll. You're not going to be like, 'Wow, I'm grazing, look at me at the vegetable restaurant, grazing . . . wow, isn't this . . . remarkable.'

"The rutabaga, which is just one of my favorite vegetables in the world, we slice very thin and we roast it down in the oven with a touch of sherry vinegar, olive oil, fresh thyme, salt and pepper. We julienne them, and it has the amazing texture of cheese and it's just awesome in salad."

Garbanzo bourdetto, tomato, mint, oregano, olives, white beet skordalia.

"In *For Your Eyes Only,* James Bond goes to Greece and he orders bourdetto. And I said, 'What the hell is that?' So I googled it and did some research. It's a casserole dish in Greece. It's very rustic, and I've really never seen it on a menu anywhere. But if James Bond can eat it, so can we.

"We're gonna do this with garbanzos cooked with tomato, white wine, peppers, onions, mint, oregano, dill. That flavor profile we've used before at Horizons and really enjoyed.... It's haunting, almost, the way they come together; the end effect is greater than the parts of those herbs.

"The really cool part about this dish is the skordalia, which is one of my favorite things in the world. It's essentially potatoes and sometimes bread, sometimes almonds, with olive oil and a touch of sherry vinegar, made into a paste. It's a Greek dip. I love it because it usually has 10 cloves of garlic in there. It makes you healthy in the wintertime, which is really nice.

"We're gonna make our skordalia with white beets instead of potatoes, a little bread and some olive oil, and it's just going to sing on top of that Greek-inspired stew underneath."

Braciole: Smoked eggplant and cauliflower, salsa verde, olive bagna cauda.

"This is one of my all-time favorite dishes I've ever done in the 17 [years] that I've been serving food to people. Number one, I love eggplant, but you've got to cook it right. What we do is to slice the eggplant really thin, paper thin, and we just give it a slight roast in the oven so it just turns translucent. It's not chewy, it's not white and gummy, it's just translucent. And we stuff it with smoked eggplant and ground-up cauliflower and wrap it up.

"This dish also has a special meaning: It's downsized from the Horizons menu into one of these medium-sized plates. At Horizons, OK, we came up with this braciole ... I loved it, but it was busier than it needed to be.

"This was our inspiration: We've got to stop when this dish was done.

"It's going to be one-note, simple brushstrokes, the way food should be. It's not going to be too busy. There won't be colorful oils or microgreens or fried leek cages or sparklers on top of it."

Feb 23, 2012
More African-Americans Turning Diets Around

"A lot of people might be very surprised at the number of African-Americans who are health-conscious and who are vegan," Evelyn Redcross said.

She wasn't kidding. I've been told, straight-faced, that "black vegans" are nonexistent, since the "veggie" thing is just spoiled white college kids acting out.

But in fact there are many reasons and rationales for eating vegan and vegetarian. Redcross believes a more health-conscious attitude in her own community is helping bring people out to the vegan brunch she and her husband, Mercer, throw nearly every Sunday at the 7165 Lounge, their banquet facility on Germantown Avenue in Mount Airy.

"Just look in the Callowhill Whole Foods," Redcross continued. "And see the percentage of African-Americans in there looking for healthier food."

"Easily 20 percent," Mercer chimed in. "And they're not there because they want to spend a lot of money on food," he said, laughing.

Stephanie Daniel, a brunch regular and tennis instructor, sees a growing trend: "More and more black people, and everyone else, want to turn their diet around."

At the brunch, there's a festive but relaxed atmosphere, with live music. Sam Lackey takes requests at the keyboard for much of the afternoon, and a band was rehearsing onstage as I arrived. The elegantly presented buffet offers a wide variety of good vegan food, all you can eat for $12.

"There's a choice of five or six items, plus a hearty salad with some serious vegetables," Evelyn Redcross explained. She noted signature dishes like "[vegan] sausage mushroom balls and sea cake—people who don't know think they're eating crab cakes—chili, lasagna, French toast, pancakes."

On my visit I also saw beans and rice, sausage and tofu scramble, and a side of collard greens.

Darrell Cuff, another brunch patron, was raving about the collards: "I'm about to go back there and get the chef and hold him down: 'What did you put in these greens?'"

Obviously, in this case, bacon, fatback and chicken stock are all absent. But the chef, Sanford "Stan" Redcross, a relative of Mercer's, said there was no big secret recipe: "Vegetable stock—that's the best you can use—and then salt and pepper to taste. A little cane sugar—evaporated cane juice."

The Lounge avoids white sugar and cooks with brown rice, relying on the freshness of the ingredients to sell the flavor.

"We wanted to introduce more people to this lifestyle," said Evelyn Redcross. "What better way than to have a kitchen and offer fresh vegan food?"

Mercer Redcross agreed: "When people are ready to listen and consider alternatives, we gotta be there with fresh food. And let them taste it." He dropped his voice to an intimate, confidential tone: "'Can you really tell the difference? Is there a big difference?' If it's marginal, then they're ready to hear what we're saying."

True to the diversity within the movement, Evelyn and Mercer came to improved eating via slightly different motives. Mercer went vegetarian over a concern for animal cruelty; Evelyn said the health aspect was what first turned her toward veganism.

The couple have two grown sons—one vegetarian, one vegan—and a daughter, Stephanie, who is making waves in national vegan social-media circles with her marketing site Vegan Mainstream.

While the Redcrosses are driven, they're not unique: Many at the Lounge noted other healthy-food spots nearby, especially the African-oriented the Nile just a few blocks down Germantown Avenue. Education is important, they agreed, but nothing compares with providing actual food.

"Talking is good," said Evelyn Redcross. "But when people can experience something new, they can change. Last week, someone I'd been dealing with on this for over a year texted me: 'I've been vegetarian for three months.'"

She smiled. "People are transitioning."

Apr 5, 2012
Vegan Food Traveler Finds Philly's among the Best

Kristin Lajeunesse can't be the only person who's ever thought of traveling the United States eating at every vegan restaurant. But she's the one who's actually doing it, in a project called "Will Travel for Vegan Food." Her journey began last fall, and in March she came through Philadelphia. I interviewed her afterward to get an outsider's perspective on our veg scene.

Q: How did this go from "crazy idea" to a reality of your daily life?

A: I was ready to start living these "dreams" I had. I left my 9-to-5 job, set up a social-media consulting business, spent a few months planning the trip and securing a van, started a Kickstarter project to help fund gas and food, and then . . . I was off!

Q: Before you got to Philly, what eateries did you find noteworthy?

A: G-Zen in Branford, Conn.; Eden Vegetarian in Bar Harbor, Maine; and Borrowed Earth Cafe in Downers Grove, Ill.

Q: How did our town's vegan offerings compare with other cities'?

A: Among the best! Hands down. Between the standouts, the overall vegan-friendliness of non-veg restaurants, and the ease of walking around (everything seemed to be within a mile of each other, which made it easy to walk/bus around), the overall experience was one of my best so far.

Q: What Philly place stands out the most for you?

A: Vedge is absolutely one of my all-time favorites of the entire road trip to date. Mostly it's the creativity that's put into each meal, as if every bite had its own pop of flavor.

Q: OK, no surprise there, but other than Vedge?

A: Blackbird Pizzeria and Grindcore House—I definitely spent the most time at both of these places. Blackbird's vegan pizza is truly one of a kind. Unique pies with crazy delicious toppings. And their cheesesteak is the best I had in all of Philly. Grindcore House was my first experience with an all-vegan coffee house. I fell in love with their mocha lattes with soy whip drizzled with chocolate syrup. So. Good. I would move to Philly for just these two places.

Q: Any surprises here?

A: A vegan restaurant that completely caught me off guard was Sprig & Vine in New Hope. The food was simply magnificent and the ambience was tip-top. And they pay attention.

Q: Did you find any common thread among Philly venues?

A: Absolutely. It had little to do with food or ambience, however. It was the sense of community and connectedness among the restaurants and overall vegan community. It was beautiful, really. I have yet to see this kind of group support anywhere else.

Mar 26, 2015
Pat's Steaks Owner: Vegan Cheesesteaks Even Better This Year

The grand finale of the 2015 Best Vegan Cheesesteak in Philly contest was a blast—a blast of very-late-winter snow!

On Friday, three hours before spring's start, Philly was covered in wet, white stuff, jamming traffic and slamming our final judging event at Weavers Way Chestnut Hill.

Two of our perennially prompt judges arrived late, as a fallen tree closed the main road from Center City, and many of those expected wound up being thwarted from attending. Still, a healthy throng of vegan and vegan-curious spectators cheered our judges (Frank Olivieri Jr., Councilwoman Cindy Bass, Dr. Ana Negron and dietitian Ed Coffin) as contest finalists Blackbird Pizzeria, Royal Tavern and Jerry's Kitchen submitted their wares.

American Vegan Society president Freya Dinshah was on hand as part of the store's celebration of FARM's Great American

Meatout, and she graciously agreed to step in and collaboratively judge with the late-arriving Coffin.

The judges chose the sandwich from Royal Tavern as top Vegan Cheesesteak, with former titleholder Blackbird taking solace in the fact that its rival won with seitan made by Blackbird's own Mark Mebus.

Olivieri, proprietor of Pat's King of Steaks, suggested that the quality of the entries had risen. "I think they all stepped up their game this year," he told me. "The sandwiches are just getting better."

Royal Tavern's Mark McKinney, who last year took second place with Cantina Dos Segundos's "vegan cheesesteak burrito," later told me that he was especially intrigued to attempt the real deal—only vegan—because "I never have had an actual Philly cheesesteak."

Was he able to definitively answer the question I always hear around this time of year: "What's a meatless, cheeseless cheesesteak made out of?"

McKinney saw it as a matter of individual taste: "Seitan is closest in texture to meat, but I have friends who swear by soy protein or portobello mushroom." He noted that three out of the five judges remarked positively on the inclusion of roasted mushrooms in Royal Tavern's entry, which "may have put me over the edge."

For those who want to try this at home, McKinney cautioned about overcooking: "Remember that [seitan and soy protein] are foods that have already been cooked, so you want to go as light as possible. Don't hammer them. Strive for a good texture."

As for the newly crowned champion himself, he says he's busy dealing with "the business [the win] is causing. We've tripled our vegan cheesesteak sales since Friday."

And the chef who put Royal Tavern, Khyber Pass, Cantina Dos Segundos and others on Philly's vegan-friendly map is prepping a new slate of plant-based treats at Triangle Tavern, set to launch in mid-April.

"Wait till you try the vegan meatballs," he promised. "And the vegan hot roast beef sandwich."

They already sound like all-time favorites. And if previous McKinney creations are any indication, it's no contest.

Jun 4, 2015
Meatless but "Meaty" Meatballs a Superior Experience

The Italian Market just marked a century in business, and it didn't get there by catering to dietary fads. The vendors' hallmark in this South Philly area is patient, high-quality craftsmanship, developed over time.

Originally established by old-world cheesemakers, butchers and sausage-grinders, and reveling in its traditional trappings, this is not where you'd look for trailblazing vegan foods.

Sure, there are scattered options: Sabrina's Cafe, after all, has competed in our vegan cheesesteak contest. And you can find Vegan Treats cookies and whoopie pies at Gleaner's Cafe or grab a vegan wrap a block east at Lyas Cafe. A selection of vegan items has, it seems, become mandatory for new Philly cafes.

But just off the corner of 9th and Christian, there's a whole 'nother level of animal-free innovation: Superior Pasta, a 67-year market fixture, since January has been rolling out vegan versions of its handmade specialties, showing how traditional food techniques can blend with 21st-century ethics, with delicious results.

Proprietor Joe Lomanno explains: "A longtime customer named Lisa [Timmons] came in all the time to get our marinara, and lots of meatballs. One time I remarked how she must love our meatballs, and she said, 'Actually I don't. They're for my husband. I'm vegan.'"

Timmons continued the tale: "I said maybe Joe should look into doing a vegan version of his celebrated meatballs, because that's their specialty, and he said he was open to it."

Next time Timmons stopped in, she was surprised to be invited to try the latest batch.

It wasn't just a thank you or a PR move—Lomanno, his son Joe Lomanno Jr. and his head pasta maker Rodger Holst had been carefully testing and retesting the vegan meatball concept, blending textured soy protein with nutritional yeast and almond milk, and finally with raw cashews, to achieve a surprisingly, almost disturbingly meaty vegan meatball.

"Rodger got excited about it," noted Lomanno Sr., "because he has a lot of vegan friends." Their feedback helped the team adjust their recipes.

And it paid off: While vegan meatballs were already available in Philly (I reviewed Ikea's at Philly.com/veganikea), Superior's fresh-made, rolled-by-hand entries have easily grabbed the title of most amazing vegan meatballs around.

The same can be said of Superior's vegan ravioli, both the "3 cheese" and porcini varieties. Lomanno chronicled the trial-and-error process for getting the perfect texture in the filling through "about five different tries," eventually achieving the desired smoothness.

"In the case of the porcini, most people would not be able to tell the difference" between the vegan and regular versions, Lomanno said, beaming. "The cheese ones are good, too, but they're not gonna fool anybody." I may not have been fooled, but I can tell you that the extensive testing paid off in another Superior product.

Having conquered ravioli, the team moved on to vegan scallopini, then spinach lasagna, which made its debut last week, another smooth and flavorful hit. Again it was the result of careful testing and modification over time. Says Joe Lomanno Jr., "The vegan mozzarella helped a great deal on that one. We tried several kinds and settled on [the brand] Daiya as the one that really worked best."

Rather than resting on his laurels, Lomanno Sr. is looking to expand both the vegan line and its availability. He's in talks with a handful of upscale grocers to carry the meatballs, for starters.

Also available is a vegan spinach pasta (the traditional recipe contains eggs), and "a vegan eggplant parm will be coming soon, but we still haven't got it right," Lomanno candidly admits, insisting that they achieve something "on a par with our wonderful regular eggplant parm."

As for longtime vegan Timmons, having gotten these meatballs rolling, she says that "now I'm inspired to do more, to speak up more" about potential vegan options in local shops.

And why not? If such a traditional bastion of time-honored quality can apply its skills to new vegan foods, what's stopping, say, your own neighborhood deli?

The plant-based treats are already garnering acclaim as people learn about them, says Lomanno. "We have vegans coming in here pretty excited, maybe because there's not a lot of this kind of food, Italian-style foods, available to them."

At the same time, he's finding some meat-eating customers picking up the new items, either to try themselves or for a family member. He cited the growing number of family celebrations involving one or two vegans. "People want to have something good to feed to a loved one that happens to eat differently," he said.

"So, however it goes, we're gonna stick with it," he explained, with a mix of compassion and shrewd business sense. "Let's face it: The vegan community is growing—and in terms of food, it's a preference based on a personal commitment. That's not gonna go away."

Nov 14, 2013

Meatless Monday Resolution—a Good First Step, But...

Depending on how you count it, Meatless Monday, endorsed by City Council this fall, is a movement that's been around for a decade—or a century.

In 2003, the Johns Hopkins Bloomberg School of Public Health Center for a Livable Future put its official stamp on Meatless Mondays—simply eating meat-free on that day to avoid the known health liabilities of meat and get more mouth-time for fruits and veggies.

But there were also "Meatless Mondays" back in World War I, launched by the United States Food Administration to conserve resources. (Animal agriculture is a notably inefficient package for nutrients.)

It was more the taking of animals' lives for our dinner plates that motivated the animal advocacy group the Humane League to push the city for its resolution.

Put together, these all make a compelling case.

Rachel Atcheson, director of the Humane League in Philly, explained that in addition to members educating their own representatives, her team worked particularly with Councilman Bill Green (who introduced the resolution) and Councilwoman Blondell Reynolds Brown. "They were key in getting other [Council members] on board," she said.

The resolution, which has no enforcement aspect, clearly appealed to Reynolds Brown, already known for her nutrition-related efforts, including a 2010 city menu-labeling law.

So will she observe Meatless Mondays herself?

"Absolutely, positively in capital letters," the Councilwoman replied, expressing a preference for "black bean soup and a nice salad" as her go-to meatless meal. She's devoted to helping constituents take charge of their eating habits.

"Obesity is a crisis in the African-American community," she noted in discussing menu labeling, but "research shows that when consumers are provided with information on the front end, they make better decisions."

So Meatless Monday lets us all take a look at what we're eating and modify it in an animal-free direction. It's a step—but how big?

In other words, maybe the resolution has no teeth, but does it have legs?

Mark McDonald, press secretary for Mayor Nutter (who was out of the country at the time), said the mayor had no Meatless Monday events on his calendar, but he reminded me that "the mayor does not eat red meat."

McDonald said the idea of a meatless day is in sync with city programs like the Healthy Corner Stores Network, which helps boost access to fresh, healthy foods.

So far, the School District of Philadelphia has no plans to implement Meatless Mondays, a spokesperson said. Atcheson has meetings scheduled with a couple charters and two suburban school districts to explore how such a program could work.

The idea is not without opposition, though.

It was no surprise that the USDA quickly retracted an endorsement in its own newsletter after howls from Big Meat. Or that Glenn Beck fears the "nanny state" running amok.

But it's also a campaign that makes some vegans queasy.

Logically, after all, if we're cutting out meat for saturated fat and cholesterol, we should be cutting out dairy. Ditto if we're concerned about livestock's contribution to climate change, or about the pain and death intrinsic to any form of animal agriculture. Why cut one "bad" thing and leave the rest untouched?

Ideologically, it seems arbitrary: Rutgers law professor Gary Francione announced "No Small, Factory-Farmed Fish Fridays" to satirize rejecting one animal product while promoting others. He suggested instead that "Vegan Monday" (or whatever day) would at least be an ethically consistent step.

In terms of day-to-day eating, though, Meatless Mondays are a doable goal for mainstream eaters and one that advocates hope will inspire further goals, whether motivated by health, environment, or animal-free concerns.

As Reynolds Brown noted, if people are coming at their food with open eyes, they're more likely to modify their habits. Among its other offerings, Meatless Monday can be a showcase for eye-opening vegan meals.

Resolutions such as this one start a much-needed and, most importantly, ongoing conversation on changing eating patterns.

So . . . go meatless! And keep going!

Aug 9, 2012
Philly Bar Scene Is Beginning to Embrace Veg-Head Customers

It wasn't that long ago that sidling up to the bar for a beer and a veggie burger was a comical incongruity. But as vegan food goes mainstream, pubs around Philly are now stepping up to serve us not just burgers but creative sandwiches and snack concoctions that often rival their meat-based mainstays.

Some intrepid pioneer had to map this territory by going out drinking all over town. I unhesitatingly volunteered.

But I couldn't pull it off alone, so I teamed up with the man who knows the ropes: [*Daily News* beer columnist] Joe Sixpack.

Through word-of-mouth and help from web sites, I had found about a dozen spots around the city with standout items. While I couldn't cover them all for this column, I did some sampling and concentrated on a core venue-hopping jaunt with Joe.

We started our journey at the place that earns the "most improved" award in terms of veggie food—Khyber Pass Pub, now a sit-down joint without live music.

OK, some people would say that's a non-improvement from the legendary, loud and lively grease-pit the Khyber used to be, but the food tips the balance.

BBQ pulled pork, fried chicken, coleslaw, Italian sausage and buttered popcorn are rendered in all-vegan versions. I particularly liked the sausage, with more fennel kick than you usually get. I mentioned my plan to stick to vegan beers, and that turned the conversation into a kind of beer summit over the question of what's practical and possible in living vegan. Joe Sixpack wrote up his own take as a separate column, but I said that with easy resources like Barnivore.com, why not go ahead with beer we can agree is vegan-friendly?

I was drinking an Allagash White, which I knew was vegan because I used to get it at Horizons, and Joe, taking off from wheat beer and white beer and why they're likely to be vegan, recommended a Franziskaner Hefelweisse, which went with both the pulled pork and sausage sandwiches perfectly.

Another place we hit that night was Cantina Dos Segundos, where tasty, crispy seitan tacos were on special. While not quite in the Khyber's league (though owned by the same folks), Dos Segundos's menu features some seitan-based options among other veg-friendly, Mexican-tinged offerings.

At The Abbaye, I had their vegan wings washed down by a Troeg's Perpetual IPA. This was the only IPA I had (I usually go a little mellower). I don't know if that was a factor, but the wings were pretty much overpowered by the beer.

In Joe's opinion, what they were missing was "bones," and he had a point. Such creations would benefit from something extra, texturally, to provide more resistance and contrast.

We closed the night out at the Standard Tap, which offered a chickpea sandwich that I was too full to try (but somehow managed to squeeze in a Victory Whirlwind Wit).

Other than that Beer Summit, I also hit Monk's Cafe for a veggie cheesesteak (vegan without cheese), West Philly's Local 44 for a seitan-pastrami Reuben, and South Philadelphia Tap Room, where I enjoyed its one-of-a-kind "vegan hoagie" along with a Kenzinger Kolsch.

That texture-rich multilayered masterpiece was the "all-around munchable" winner from my own travels. But you may have your own to add to the list.

The important thing is to recognize Philly as not just a great beer town—but a great pub-food town.

Jun 27, 2013
Vegan Pizza's So Hot, It Has a Day

It's no surprise to find a veggie burger on a diner menu. Nowadays, any place with burgers that lacks a veggie option is self-consciously retro.

Surprising to some, though, is that the same thing is now happening with pizza. To celebrate Vegan Pizza Day—a national event taking place this Saturday—let's survey the scene.

Just a few years ago, vegan pizza in Philly was as scarce as a medium-rare unicorn, but today you can find it at a dozen places, as more businesses apply the veggie-burger principle (don't give a party of people that includes a vegan a reason to go elsewhere).

Take Frankford Avenue's Pizza Brain, which opened with terrific hype as the Pizza Museum, based on an info-taining decor that celebrates everything pizza-related. Who could claim comprehensiveness without including a vegan variety?

I stopped by recently and found its offering to be delicious. It's their regular crust and tangy sauce with Daiya cheese, to which you can add veggies or whatever, though I stuck with the plain cheese because, you know, science.

The smallest option, a personal pizza (no vegan slices available yet), seemed sized for a bigger person—which indeed I was by the time I left.

There was no room for dessert. Which was sad, since Little Baby's Ice Cream (with plenty of vegan flavors) has a stand attached to the restaurant.

Pizza Brain joins stalwarts like Manayunk's Couch Tomato, chains like Slice and newcomers like PWS on Powelton Avenue as mainstream pizza joints that have included plant-based eaters in their business plan.

The normalizing of vegan pizza is partly due to the foresight of local pioneers like Ed's in West Philly and, of course, Blackbird Pizzeria off South Street.

And then there's Vegan Pizza Day. Founded by a California blogger and a Chicago vegan-cheese company, the holiday is now in its third year and gathering steam. No parades are scheduled yet, but you can celebrate by eating at one of these venues—or by making your own at home, thanks to recent vegan-pizza lines from Tofurky, Daiya and American Flatbread.

However you slice it, this event underscores the fact that vegan pizza has arrived, with tasty cheese that melts and/or a variety of healthful veggie toppings.

Speaking of toppings, Blackbird, already a beloved institution, continues to push the vegan-pizza concept in fun directions. Owner Mark Mebus says he'll be celebrating the day by previewing some of the new varieties on his upcoming revamped menu.

It's worth noting that all-vegan spots like Blackbird have helped blaze the trail into which nonvegan venues are now tiptoeing. Stop in for a slice, and taste the future!

Another place you can do so this Saturday is Govinda's Gourmet to Go. That's right, the venerable Broad-and-South fast-food spot is about to start doing pizza!

Owner Hari (a.k.a. Howard Brown) says that vegan pizza will be added to the regular menu in July, and on Saturday's special occasion you can try out a slice or two. Tell 'em "V for Veg" sent you!

Even if you can't get to any of these locations, remember: Your neighborhood pizza place can and should make tomato pies. (Hold the sprinkled Parmesan!)

Vegan Pizza Day might be a good time to suggest adding vegan cheese on one. Come on, it's a pizza party!

Don't get me wrong: I'm not saying that it's the case right now that any pizza joint you walk into will have vegan pizza on the menu.

All I'm saying is that it will be.

May 16, 2013
Magic Chefs
At Vedge, Nothing That Grows Goes Unimproved

Rich Landau is a magician. What other explanation is there for the amazing tricks he pulls off with vegetables?

Fingerling Potatoes with Creamy Worcestershire Sauce? Roasted Cauliflower with Black Vinegar and Kimchi Cream? In every case, the veggies retain their flavor essence while surprising and delighting. It's a culinary feat that seems beyond mere mortals.

And it's no fluke: From the "Food of the Future" days of Horizons Cafe in Willow Grove to the last days of "Modern Vegan Cuisine" Horizons off South Street, and now their latest project—the sophisticated "vegetable restaurant" Vedge—Landau and his wife and partner, Kate Jacoby, have consistently wowed even the carnivore crowd with vegan creations that prompt the awestruck "how do they do it?" of a magic show.

Through its example and influence, Horizons—which opened in 1994 in Willow Grove, then relocated to Queen Village from 2006 to 2011—helped remap Philly as a vegan-restaurant town. Now Vedge, which opened in 2011, has helped push vegetable-centered cuisine into the mainstream, landing on GQ's 12 Best Restaurants of 2013 list.

"Chef Richard Landau's staff must include a benevolent gremlin or a fairy godmother who sprinkles magic dust over the pots and the pans," theorized GQ's Alan Richman, who seemed more than a little bewitched. "I had no idea so much flavor could be delivered without butter, cream, milk, eggs and other kitchen staples."

Now they're pulling back the curtain with the new cookbook *Vedge: 100 Plates Large and Small That Redefine Vegetable Cooking*. Out in July from The Experiment, it takes curious amateur chefs backstage to see how the magic works. But, as with any magic trick, the explanation may be deceptively simple.

"Let the ingredients speak," Landau reiterated last week. "Put vegetables on the pedestal, embellish them, enhance them, do something that no one's ever done before—but let people know that it is what it is.

"I'm not going to take carrots and make them into sausage or foams or make a caramel-carrot cage out of them. I want you to know you're eating carrots, but I am also going to challenge myself to spice them in a way that the spices don't become the first thing you taste on your palate. You should taste carrots first, then the spices, but I also wanted to prepare them in a way that's like, 'Oh I never thought of that.'"

The new cookbook applies this treatment to a massive number of vegetables.

"We tried to find one recipe for every single vegetable," Landau said. "The only vegetable I know, off the top of my head, that isn't in there is artichokes."

To my mock horror, he added, "I know! They're just a pain in the ass to prep."

Jacoby added, "We even thought of structuring the book like 'Ingredients' or 'Root Vegetables' or 'Potatoes' or whatever, but that's not quite how we approach food. We think of flavors first."

Reproducing flavors developed in a well-staffed commercial kitchen for dishes that home chefs can manage was part of the trick here. But the book does that—and with the restaurant's signature cocktails and creative desserts, too. Both categories are Jacoby's specialty.

While we get tipped to some secrets—many passages share welcome wisdom on spice combining and judicious substitution—some magic stays at Vedge.

"Some things you not only can't 'translate,' but I can't even make them at home myself," Landau laughed. "The eggplant bracciole just kind of snuck in there because I found a way to do a version of it at home. Not the restaurant version, which is hours and hours of very precise prep, but it will be close, and something people can do in their own kitchen."

Landau sees this process as part of his mission to help people re-examine what they're eating and why.

He recalled that before the first of the two Horizons cookbooks—*Horizons: The Cookbook* (Book Publishing Co., 2005) and *Horizons: New Vegan Cuisine* (Horizons, 2007)—people would often say, "Wow, if I could cook this way, I'd be vegan." But there's an implicit flip side here: "Since I can't cook like this, I'm going to eat dead animal flesh."

Since "we have to sleep at night," Landau continued, there was "definitely a cause behind that [Horizons] cookbook. We wanted to demystify vegan cuisine, to break down the barriers."

The *Vedge* cookbook addresses the all-too-common mentality of "just got all these veggies at the CSA. Better boil some water and cook 'em."

"No!" Landau exclaimed. "Everyone goes right for that, they start blanching them or they roast them. Well, here's some ideas that you can do where vegetables are not just a side dish anymore—maybe they can be more of the forefront of the meal, maybe they can really shine for you."

That said, the animal-free ethos is still a key motivator. Referencing the current "farm-to-table" vogue, Jacoby noted that "there's a lot of attention now to food and its production. And when you think about where food comes from, it's a whole lot nicer to think about vegetable gardens than about slaughterhouses."

Landau and Jacoby are striving for nothing less than remaking the American palate. It's an almost unthinkable task, but who else could get those of us who hated Brussels sprouts as kids (show of hands?) to voluntarily, eagerly order them for dinner? (One way: Try the recipe on page 25 for Shaved Brussels Sprouts with Whole-Grain Mustard Sauce.)

Besides, this team has not only its track record to consider, but recent developments that are spreading Vedge-consciousness beyond Philly.

At the turn of the year, Williams-Sonoma launched three Vedge-branded sauces, bringing the Vedge magic to America's kitchens. Landau and Jacoby have made key forays—cooking for Bill Clinton at a New York City fundraiser and sharing their skills at acclaimed Laloux for February's Montreal en Lumiere festival. All this after being the first vegan restaurant invited to showcase at Manhattan's legendary James Beard House.

More big things are in the offing, with a Los Angeles edition of Vedge getting closer to realization. Landau and Jacoby head out west in a couple of weeks to check out potential locations.

Meanwhile, look for them soon on your TV screen, in major magazines and at key big-city dinners and events as the cookbook promotion revs into high gear.

As the accolades roll in, Landau and Jacoby keep pushing forward, creating magical new combinations with nothing up their sleeves but produce.

Although the "farm-to-table" fad may fade, Landau is confident that the plant-based approach that the *Vedge* cookbook promotes has staying power.

"Vegetables will never go out of style. They're food. They've been growing in the ground as long as humans have walked the planet. That's what we eat, and this is a great new way to discover it."

Jul 10, 2014
Another Philadelphia First: Birthplace of U.S. Veganism

Philadelphia is the "birthplace of America"—and of veganism in the United States!

Hyperbole? Not really—here's why.

The American Vegan Society, founded in 1960 by H. Jay Dinshah, in Malaga, NJ, is at the root of nearly every major development in the spread of vegan living on this continent. And Dinshah was standing at the corner of Front and Venango streets in Philly when he decided to go vegan.

A new book edited by Jay's daughter, Anne Dinshah, *Powerful Vegan Messages: Out of the Jungle for the Next Generation* (American

Vegan Society), has the story: That corner was the location of the Cross Brothers slaughterhouse, which Jay and his brother Nosheran toured in 1957 to settle an argument about whether their vegetarianism was truly ethical.

Leaving this facility, having seen dairy cows slaughtered, and realizing that dairy and meat were part of the same industry, Dinshah stood on that corner and vowed to go vegan and fight—nonviolently—for a vegan world.

He launched the AVS, the foundation on which dozens of well-known animal-advocacy groups have built since then.

Unlike in the United Kingdom, where the first Vegan Society was started by Donald and Dorothy Watson and others in 1944, vegans were hard to find in the U.S. in the pre-Internet 1960s. Dinshah and his wife, Freya, helped to create a vegan network via newsletters and lecture tours.

Jay spoke on "dynamic harmlessness," or proactive nonviolence, and behind the scenes Freya handled all the food issues. In 1965, after several coast-to-coast tours, she had gathered enough recipes, plus her own veganized versions of family favorites, to publish the first "vegan"-titled cookbook in the U.S., *The Vegan Kitchen* (American Vegan Society).

Anne Dinshah's mission with *Powerful Vegan Messages* (americanvegan.org) was to update and package Jay's pioneering writings for today's world.

Many of the topics he tackled masterfully, from animal agriculture's degradation of the planet to the impossibility of living "100 percent vegan," are still "introduced" as controversies by vegan writers who should know better.

A half-century before the ersatz "paleo" craze, Dinshah called for a higher standard than that of our ancestors in his essay collection *Out of the Jungle* (American Vegan Society): Claiming "civilization" as the hallmark of our species, we can't then cite "the law of the jungle" as an excuse to perpetuate unnecessary cruelty and violence toward our fellow sentient beings.

"How is it," he asked, "that we claim to be the highest type of creature, yet act in a barbaric manner that would shame any reasonably decent denizen of the jungle? Do we not make our civilized world a more terribly cruel and unjust place than any natural jungle?"

Powerful Vegan Messages weaves chapters and passages from this and other Dinshah writings with perspectives from Anne and dozens of other prominent vegan advocates who work to convey the wide-ranging influence and inspirational humility of the man who kick-started American veganism at Front and Venango.

That slaughterhouse, of course, has another claim to fame: In 1962, Joe Frazier got a job there and practiced boxing by hitting sides of beef—a detail Sylvester Stallone later used in *Rocky* (UA, 1976). And, yes, that scene of Rocky punching cow carcasses was shot at Cross Brothers.

Philly loves Rocky, of course, as an underdog who stuck to his dream to go the distance in an epic fight. Mainstreaming the vegan idea in America is a fight that Jay Dinshah promised to stick to until the day he died, and he did.

Back in 1960, the vegan idea was less than a blip in popular consciousness, but Dinshah worked tirelessly for this underdog ideology. Today, "vegan" is a household word, gaining more traction every day both in Philly and across the continent, while in Malaga, under the direction of Freya Dinshah, the AVS furthers its work of education and outreach.

Meanwhile, with constant PR "black eyes" like the current salmonella outbreak in chicken; with now-indisputable links between processed meats and cancer, and between animal agriculture and climate change; with per capita meat and milk consumption falling and beef prices hitting new heights, the longtime "champ" may be on the ropes.

And thanks to Jay Dinshah, the true underdogs—the billions of innocent animals whose lives are stolen by our mindless eating habits—now have more than a fighting chance.

THE BIG PICTURE

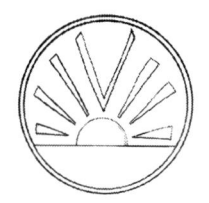

Apr 5, 2014
Yes, *Noah* Is Totally Vegan Propaganda

How do you make a movie involving an ark filled with animals that doesn't use a single real animal? My interest in Darren Aronofsky's *Noah* (Paramount) was piqued when I heard this detail about its production, then heightened when I learned the spread for the movie's premiere was vegan.

When I saw some grumbling about the vegan director ticking people off by injecting such elements into the telling of this hallowed story, I had to check it out, and I'm back to report that yes, *Noah* is indeed, gopherwood-wall-to-gopherwood-wall, vegan propaganda.

As a work of art, it probably misses being a "great" movie, saddled as it is with "big-budget Hollywood spectacle" tropes. It is, however, definitely a milestone in blockbuster veganism, in mainstreaming the vegan idea, weaving it through related issues—justice, faith, sacrifice, masculinism, militarism, climate change, violence, nonviolence and storytelling—that make for a moving and thought-provoking experience for anyone who's paying attention.

The stakes are set in the film's opening minute: Among quick clips accompanying the story of the Fall we see a hand reaching for an apple—except the apple is beating, like a heart, both visually and audibly. This is a jaw-dropping visual and philosophical mashup, implying that the real "forbidden fruit," the arrogant behavior that led to our current fallen condition, was killing and eating animals once we knew the difference between good and evil.

Indeed, Noah and his family are introduced gathering berries and other plant foods, as Noah admonishes them "we collect only what we need." An ecological ethic, this is also a vegan one: We need to eat plants to survive, but we don't need to eat animals. For the wisest member of the family, berry-eating turns into an epic, life-affirming quest, as if to underscore that literal fruit was not forbidden, and what was "forbidden" was not, in fact, a fruit.

The violence inherent in the opening hand-on-heart image is followed immediately by that of Cain slaying Abel—connecting man's violence vs. animals to his violence vs. himself—and Aronofsky "adapts" the somewhat contrary element of Cain, the killer, being a vegetarian by completely omitting it. (He also conveniently omits God's explicit allowance of nonveganism after the flood, a passage that would be dissonant if included, but which does show that through this portion of the Biblical story, Noah must have been vegan.)

Early on, Noah's values and his sense of justice are expressed in his bid to save a hunted, mortally wounded animal, at which point he has to explain to his surprised children that some people actually eat animals—because "they think it makes them stronger." This immediately follows Noah delivering an ass-whooping to three homicidal meat-eaters at once, showing he's plenty strong without consuming flesh.

Meanwhile, Tubal-cain's clan of meat-eaters follow their ethos to its logical extreme. They terrorize, capture, subjugate and eat animals, and likewise they terrorize, capture and subjugate people—and yes, eat that flesh too. Again human-on-human carnage is equated with that of human on animal.

This meat-eating version of the Fall is rendered more explicit later when Tubal-cain talks Noah's rebellious son Ham into eating another "forbidden fruit": some of the anesthetized animals that are on board. (His doing so, I'm betting, is repulsive to most moviegoers, for reasons they might want to examine.) Tubal-cain rationalizes his food choice by exalting human supremacy—our outpacing the Creator by forcing animals to "serve us."

Tubal-cain serves as an at times too-convenient mouthpiece to express the twisted "logic" of animal subjugation. This speech goes a bit over the top on the evil-meter (and movie-meter) but he's not always cranked up to 11, and in fact is most disturbing when his words echo mainstream present-day discourse. His equating "being a man" with being willing to kill another man (which, again, he underscores by killing another animal) is almost indistinguishable from, and thus a poignant parody of, the might-makes-right "manly" garbage that young boys are fed 24/7 by nearly every culture on the planet.

One last Fall connection is the snakeskin (from the Snake itself), brought forward as a relic of patriliny. It's no accident that this patriarchal signifier is, at the end, applied for the first time to females. Tubal-cain's macho exceptionalism has been eradicated, and it is women who have helped to accomplish that, setting the stage for a new, more nurturing humanity going forward.

Finally, if anyone missed the point of the human/animal equation, Aronofsky shows us footage of animal families while Noah's daughter-in-law Ila explicitly straightens him out about the choice between killing vs. love—a choice, we're given to understand, that each of us has to make, using our (accursed) knowledge of the difference between doing good and doing wrong.

This casts straight back to the heart/apple image, and the story's climax casts forward to another Genesis story, inverting it as well. Through these echoes, congruence and foreshadowing, Aronofsky has done something more radical and subversive than most of the film's protesters even get: With this one iconic Biblical tale as a springboard, he's illuminated all of Genesis—all of our stories, in fact, about why we are who we are—asking how best we turn our most deeply held values and beliefs into action.

This questioning is spurred by the risky move of turning Noah unsympathetic as he becomes more invested in his dogmatic interpretation of his mission, and more seemingly wrongheaded: Does he really understand what the Creator wants, or has he become an unreliable narrator? I was unsettled by this turn myself, but it pays off—both in setting up the story's climax and in warning all of us—vegans very much included—that you can have all the truth in the world on your side and still err if you push it to an extreme that lacks compassion.

As mentioned, the vegan imperative is artfully woven into other themes—this isn't the only message in the film, just the predominant one. Many reviews point to the obvious parallel with our climate-change crisis and the need for serious environmentalism, usually throwing in the be-nice-to-animals thing as a mere example of *Noah*'s "green" ethic. This is looking through the lens from the wrong side: Aronofsky makes clear that the first step, not the last, to balancing our relationship with the world is to address our relationship to animals and to seek justice there just as we seek it among ourselves.

He also indicates that the question of how to do so transcends that of whether morality is backed up by an actual deity: Noah asks the heavens for a sign that he's released from the responsibility of a decision he doesn't want to make. But he doesn't get a sign. The decision turns out to really be up to him.

He has to choose between good and evil on his own. And that's what Aronofsky is suggesting that we all have to do, every time we pick up a fork.

Oct 5, 2015
Eating Vegan Saves
The Martian—and Us?

For the first time in a long, long, long time, I went to see a Hollywood movie on its opening weekend: *The Martian* (Fox).

Little did I know that a) I would be one of many helping push the box office to an epic, almost record-breaking weekend, or b) I'd have to write about it here.

The little I did know was from *Daily News* movie critic Gary Thompson, who told me it was "a sneaky vegan movie" on his way to submitting his review to the paper. And indeed, about the titular hero, an astronaut (Matt Damon) stranded on Mars during a storm when he's mistakenly thought to be dead, Thompson observes:

> We almost don't notice that he survives as a composting vegan who lives on organic produce, solar panels and EVs. Scott's point, I think, is not to show that man can survive on Mars, but that we can survive on Earth (note how Scott uses the movie's signature visual—a sprout poking its head through the soil).

Resigned to await the next Mars mission years away, Damon's Mark Watney stretches the leftover food rations by burying whole potatoes in Martian soil mixed with the astronauts' carefully preserved bodily waste.

He's forced to do this because—even though six people could theoretically have become stranded for an indefinite time at the Martian outpost, and even though Damon's character seems able to find any possible gewgaw or gadget he needs (including a ginormous supply of duct tape), and even though Watney is a botanist—the inventory for this Mars mission seems to not include any seeds for food.

The flip side of Watney's positive ingenuity in making food grow on Mars seems a weakness of NASA's planning: Why, you have to wonder, didn't the brilliant minds planning the mission think of this key potentially lifesaving inclusion (an extremely small and lightweight add-on compared to the quantities of luxuries shown) prior to lift-off? What was the staff botanist there for, anyway—to test the growth of long-stemmed roses?

Maybe the answer is that in this movie NASA is stuck in the same retro mindset as some laypeople I've heard remark that if and when we try to colonize Mars, we'll need to bring animals so the long-term inhabitants can have "high-quality protein." (Hey, you know what's a complete protein? Potatoes.)

Hopefully the millions who saw the movie this weekend will agree that the notion of food animals in space is patently idiotic, right? I mean, we've just watched scientists painstakingly inventory and jettison every possible gram of excess weight in order to gain propulsive power. Tossing food animals into the mix means the trip would either take longer—which would require more food rations—or eat up more precious fuel.

It's more than that, though: Live animals would require huge amounts of additional food brought along—or able to be grown—in order to even survive long enough to get to Mars. And the only advantage conferred is a psychological one—tons of biomass to deliver the same "earthly comfort" factor as, say, Commander Lewis's entire library of '70s disco, which fits on a microchip. Put simply, the math doesn't add up.

So if and when a real Martian mission happens—and the movie self-consciously serves as a cheerleader for this—I'm confident our real-world NASA will have thought this through and will prioritize health and survivability over blind tradition.

But what of that second layer Thompson mentioned? Here on Earth, the human race is Watney, facing a ticking clock with our ability to creatively and efficiently use the resources at hand determining the difference between survival and extinction. And setting aside its ethics—or lack thereof—the raising of animals for food is a grossly inefficient luxury that our species is going to need to grow out of sooner than later.

We should take Scott's message to heart, then, and act as though we were "The Martian," looking at how we can get the most benefit from the stuff at hand. Compared to Mark Watney, we have tons more fertile soil, fresh regenerating water, a greater variety of seeds and a slightly more relaxed timeline for shifting our eating entirely to plant foods.

One thing he had, but we don't, is a backup planet.

(*Vegetarian Voice* **Magazine, 2002**)
Once Upon a Crime
Animal Characters and Meat-Eating in Kids' Books

In the last scene of *Through the Looking Glass,* the trouble starts when Alice is introduced to her food, a mutton chop.

> "You look a little shy: let me introduce you to that leg of mutton," said the Red Queen. "Alice—Mutton: Mutton—Alice." The leg

of mutton got up in the dish and made a little bow to Alice; and Alice returned the bow, not knowing whether to be frightened or amused.

"May I give you a slice?" she said.

"Certainly not," the Red Queen said, very decidedly: "it isn't etiquette to cut any one you've been introduced to. Remove the joint!" And the waiters carried it off, and brought a large plum pudding in its place.

"I won't be introduced to the pudding, please," Alice said rather hastily, "or we shall get no dinner at all."

But the Queen insists on introducing them, and things escalate from there: Alice's defiance leads to an all-out banquet-table brawl.

Still, who can blame her? Being "introduced" to something you're supposed to eat brings up a stark paradox for children, and it doesn't help that what they are taught to eat—animals—are also often the main characters in stories that are read to them.

When kids come to know animal characters as intelligent, social beings with individual interests, there are inevitably going to be flash points here and there where the reality of animals as food intrudes and has to be explained away—or dealt with.

Earlier in the same book, Lewis Carroll treads similar ground in the famous poem "The Walrus and the Carpenter"—two characters who convince a bunch of credulous oysters to follow them to a secluded spot where the Walrus says,

"Now, if you're ready, Oysters dear,
We can begin to feed."
"But not on us!" the Oysters cried,
Turning a little blue.
"After such kindness, that would be
A dismal thing to do!"

"The night is fine," the Walrus said.
"Do you admire the view?"

This tragicomic moment is a singsong version of one of the darkest aspects of raising animals for food—treating them as family, teaching them to trust their caretakers, who then turn on them and kill them. Carroll boiled that dynamic down to a few words and even included the attitude of deep, fingers-in-ears denial that we must maintain to keep this vile institution going—especially over audible protests from its victims.

Then Carroll pushes it further, as the Walrus repents for this, while the Carpenter remains unmoved:

"It seems a shame," the Walrus said,
"To play them such a trick,
After we've brought them out so far,
And made them trot so quick!"
The Carpenter said nothing but
"The butter's spread too thick!"

Upon hearing this, Alice tries to determine which of the characters is less at fault in their treachery. But her answers are constantly confounded by additional incriminating information on the part of one character or the other from Tweedledum and Tweedledee: The Walrus was weeping but eating more than the Carpenter, while the latter, anyway, was eating as many as he could. Thus Carroll, no vegetarian, leaves the issue as an unsolvable riddle best left alone. Other works, however, confront humans' exploitation of animals head-on.

Probably the book that goes most overboard with this is *Black Beauty*. What opens as an animal autobiography—life seen through the eyes of another creature—soon turns into a single-minded polemic against the bearing rein, a (now obsolete) fixture that caused horses pain and struggle for the sake of fashion. One can easily imagine a through line from this "innocent" classic to the revolution wrought by the oppressed in *Animal Farm.*

Also polemical, in spurts, is *Doctor Doolittle,* the veterinarian who can understand animals' speech. He goes on about the cruelty of putting big cats in zoos until he's worked himself into a fury—then sits down to a breakfast of sausage and bacon. Throughout his adventures there's an odd admixture of these elements, challenging one institution while silently engaging in another, and very little in between.

As far as timeless classics go, probably the two that loom largest in any consideration of animal sentience are the *Wizard of Oz* series and *The Chronicles of Narnia,* which share odd correspondences. Launched exactly 50 years apart (1900, 1950), both series feature brave lions, accidental portals, wicked witches, intrepid girl heroes, powerful magic and, of course, talking animals.

In Oz, their talking isn't that noteworthy, since just about everything—sawhorses, trees, pieces of fine china—seems capable of speech. But in Narnia, talking is a matter of life and death—literally. *The Last Battle* is set in motion by the beating of a talking horse. Not a regular horse as someone here might ride or beat—of which there are also plenty in Narnia—but one that talks and is therefore almost human.

You see, while all creatures in Oz are conscious, speech-endowed individuals, Narnia has both talking beasts and "Dumb Beasts." The former are on exactly the same moral plane as people, but the latter are perfectly fine to kill for food, clothing or sport.

The kids who are constantly traveling through Narnia usually subsist on meat from one "Dumb Beast" or another. But in *The Silver Chair,* three characters are happily eating venison when they overhear their captors and realize the stag they're eating was a *talking* stag. All become nauseous. The native Narnian feels "as you would feel if you found you had eaten a baby."

C. S. Lewis creates two explicit classes of animals in Narnia—one blessed by God (who is, in this case, a carnivore) and the other completely forsaken to be used/abused for whatever purpose, an essential moral distinction based on accident of birth.

Oz plays off of the whole carnivore concept—and specifically in reference to eating babies—with an apparently vegetarian character, the Hungry Tiger, who would like nothing more than "a couple of fat babies" to eat, but is too conscience-stricken to ever do so, as he constantly reminds everyone. Meanwhile, the kids traveling through Oz almost always manage to subsist on a vegetarian diet.

True, Baum's Oz books, with the exception of *The Emerald City of Oz,* lack Narnia's pulse-quickening end-of-the-world urgency, drama and blood, but hey, blood isn't everything.

Lewis's animals are part of a tradition of British kid lit (see Tess Cosslett's *Talking Animals in British Children's Fiction* for more) that ranges beyond our topic. While Beatrix Potter's quaint tales, like Thornton Burgess's *Old Mother West Wind* series, present daily lives of animals who can expect to be preyed upon by other animals they know by name, humans (McGregor excepted) are utterly marginal to these plots.

Lesser examples of human/animal drama are too numerous to list, but are especially visible in those works picked up by Disney. In such classics as *Bambi* and *Dumbo,* the "realistic" (they don't wear clothes) young animal is painfully, forcibly separated from his mother by humans exploiting animals for recreation. Both institutions, hunting and circuses, are presented as an unchanging given that these "realistic" animals have to accept: Bambi never plots to turn the tables on the hunters, and while Dumbo raises a brief ruckus, he sticks with the circus. Animals' lives, in other words, can be ruined by humans' thoughtlessness, and there's not much the animals can do about it. They gotta be realistic!

Similarly, in *Finding Nemo,* the title fish is cruelly imprisoned in a dentist's office fish tank. And *Babar*'s mother is also killed by a hunter, though he doesn't qualify as "realistic" due to his pronounced desire to assimilate into human culture.

In *Mrs. Frisby and the Rats of NIMH*, though, the rats go through an evolution from dumb animals to genius super-rats and take on many aspects of human culture while planning their own agrarian utopia. The overheard humans' talk of rats as undifferentiated vermin contrasts throughout with the complex characters we've met.

But even with its subtle argument against vivisection, *Mrs. Frisby* doesn't set the rats in revolt against the humans; they, like Nemo, are just trying to get away.

There's one classic in which challenging the system looms large, kicking the book off in its first moments. *Charlotte's Web* opens with Fern running to stop her father from killing the pig she will wind up naming Wilbur.

Few children's books are so transparent about the gut-level human reaction to the notion of needlessly killing animals as this book's first couple pages. "This is the most terrible case of injustice I ever heard of," Fern protests, after declaring a moral equivalence between the pig's life and her own.

From there, however, E. B. White chooses to develop the story more subtly: Wilbur, like Alice's mutton, is constantly "introduced" to his would-be consumers by Charlotte's web messages. "Some Pig" points him out as a unique individual, and her further epithets continually strive to keep Wilbur a unique enough celebrity that he will not be killed by a system that—now that Fern's stopped paying attention—seems unassailable.

White was content to raise the question of animal personhood, putting talking animals in the midst of an explicitly meat-eating human world, confronting the issue without deriving an ultimate moral about it. Less subtle and in ways more satisfying in this regard is Dick King-Smith, whose animals often challenge the order of things and win over human converts.

Babe is, of course, the pig who helps humanize his farmer by successfully communicating with sheep—and herding them. But there's also Babe's cousin *Ace,* who learns to communicate on a yes-no basis with his farmer and winds up moving into his house. It's during one of Ace's long afternoons watching television that he stumbles onto a documentary on meat production and has an epiphany (shared by his young readers) about the terrible reality of most pigs' lives.

Though Farmer Hoggett and Farmer Tubbs don't turn vegetarian, the pigman in *Pigs Might Fly* practically does, renouncing ham sandwiches after witnessing the hero's bravery during a flood. And in *Martin's Mice,* the titular cat actually gives up mice—the new Hungry Tiger challenging not just our convention of meat-eating but its assumed place as a "natural, necessary" act.

In Roald Dahl's *The Magic Finger,* animal-consciousness becomes human-on-human retribution. A girl who hates her neighbors' boorish hunting parties ("I can't stand hunting. I just can't *stand* it. It doesn't seem right to me that men and boys should kill animals just for the fun they get out of it") zaps their whole family into birds—so they can experience the hunt from the other side. Another polemic in the strictest sense, I guess, but here it's mitigated by Dahl's whimsical storytelling prowess.

Dahl was famously anti-television, but the reality is that nowadays more kids are getting their animal-ethics lessons from Ronald McDonald than, say, Black Beauty or Charlotte. Let's face it: Movies may be the next best hope in teaching kids empathy for animals.

Babe: Pig in the City, the sequel, lacked some of the straightforward charm of *Babe,* but warped movie conventions to deliver important messages (no animal, no matter how small or how threatening, should be allowed to die unnecessarily). And in *WALL-E,* note that the two lead robots recognize each other's personhood in their respective kindness to a cockroach.

If movies are the next generation of classics for kids, let's get with it and look for teachable moments where we find them.

Popcorn is vegan; Milk Duds are not.

Op-Ed, Apr 21, 2015

On Earth Day, Chew on These Nutty Facts

On Earth Day, there are those who get into celebrating the planet and tweaking our lifestyle for the common good, and there are those who don't.

Those who don't sometimes make good points about home recycling bins as mere spit in the ocean of vast industrial pollution, and other times indulge in stubborn ear-plugging accompanied by magical and/or wishful thinking.

To all of us who recognize a scientifically credible threat, the head-in-sand position can be frustrating, and we might roll our eyes at its ridiculousness. Yet, even among the environmentally serious, there's a split between those who acknowledge scientific, quantifiable facts and those who go for, well, ear-plugging accompanied by magical and/or wishful thinking.

Let's talk about almonds! That's the consensus, after all, on California's epic drought and the measures recommended to combat it: Taking shorter showers is nothing compared to the almond industry's massive water use, consuming a full 10 percent of the state's water.

So, almonds are what we should really be talking about, right?

Well, they're a thirsty crop, but nothing like meat and dairy, which consume a full 47 percent of the state's water, according to a Pacific Institute report on California's "Water Footprint." Put another way: Per calorie, beef uses more than twice as much water as almonds. No matter how you slice it, meat is by far the bigger water-waster. How prominently have you seen this mentioned in water-crisis coverage?

It's not just almonds and water—the same skewed focus holds in many sectors. Quinoa production's good-news/bad-news for local economies made headlines, but not the analogous effect of animal agriculture—most starving children, after all, live in countries whose crops go to feed animals eaten by Westerners. And we hear a lot about palm-oil production resulting in the loss of rain forest, while five times as much rain forest is lost to animal agriculture.

Fracking is an eco-problem because it produces methane (almost exactly the same amount nationally as does animal agriculture) while both consuming and polluting water (as does livestock production, only more so). Climate-change discussions center on fossil-fuel alternatives—while animal agriculture is, at the least, a larger factor than all human transportation, and by some credible estimates larger than all other factors combined.

In view of public-health concerns, parents refusing vaccines for their children are vilified by parents stuffing their children and themselves with meat and dairy. Yet, in addition to meat's proven individual health risks, factory farms' casual daily use of antibiotics is driving us toward a future when antibiotics will be useless—all as 23,000 people annually are dying from new "superbugs" (CDC: Antibiotic Resistance Threats in the United States, 2013).

In almost any comparison of plant foods to animal foods, the latter are both more resource-heavy on the uptake and more Earth-unfriendly on the outflow. The only case-by-case question is whether they're just somewhat worse (as, say, cow's milk is vs. almond milk) or, more often, worse by orders of magnitude.

Thing is, most of us don't like looking at or talking about meat and dairy's origins, and opt for ear-plugging and magical/wishful thinking ("humane slaughter," anyone?) rather than tackling the most germane problems.

It's true that Earth-friendly lifestyle changes are a challenge. As mentioned, individual actions seem small compared with the big picture. But eating vegan is one change that trades the least pain (read: inconvenience) for the most gain. And it's a change that can be implemented society-wide cheaply and relatively quickly as compared with the schedule for altering our basic technological infrastructure.

Any of us who take science seriously, whether or not we're ready to drop animal foods right now, should be candidly evaluating and discussing this global polluter and leading climate-change factor.

There is, at least, a certain internal logic to pretending that "global warming" is a vast conspiracy and that we should keep everything as is.

But acknowledging the urgency of the threat and then failing to take a clear look at the most efficient, cost-effective alternatives?

That's just nuts.

(*Vegetarian Voice* Magazine, 2005)
The Decline and Fall of Human Supremacy

From antiquity up to a few hundred years ago, it was understood by nearly all human beings that the sun revolved around the earth. This made sense because, as we were the center of consciousness, creation and the universe itself, the cosmos should logically be set up as a backdrop to humanity. Thinking otherwise was heresy for some and discouraged for all.

It was a huge paradigm shift when our earth was shown to have something other than a starring role in the grand scheme, and is to some extent still being played out. The current orthodoxy is that although we were placed on an out-of-the-way planet nowhere near the center of our run-of-the-mill galaxy, our species is still the be-all and end-all of creation, or at least, failing that, of consciousness.

Now, within the last few decades, our mantra "that's what separates us from the animals," or what I call "human supremacy," has been assailed by new science on animal behavior. Within even the last couple of years this credo has been forced to stake out more complex positions on higher ground as the floodwaters of reality have swamped our previous outposts.

Tool Time

Since the dawn of time, we were supposedly the only animals with a real language. By the 20th century that notion was already discredited, and our claim to distinction became "Man the Tool-Maker." First we were the only animals that used tools, then when that was knocked down, the only animal that made tools. With documentary evidence of chimpanzees fashioning and using termite-scooping tools in rotting logs, that fell by the wayside as well.

It's a good thing the defenders of unique humanity didn't loudly proclaim that they might have tools, but we have entire *tool kits,* because it's just come to light that certain chimps also use multiple self-fashioned tools on a given job. "Using infrared, motion-triggered video cameras," *National Geographic* reported, "researchers have documented how chimpanzees in the Republic of Congo use a variety of tools to extract termites from their nests."

"The new video cameras revealed chimps using one short stick to penetrate the aboveground mounds and then a 'fishing probe' to extract the termites," the story continued. "For subterranean nests the chimps use their feet to force a larger 'puncturing stick' into the earth, drilling holes into termite chambers, and then a separate fishing probe to harvest the insects. Often the chimps modified the fishing probe, pulling it through their teeth to fray the end like a paintbrush. The frayed edge was better for collecting the insects." Pat Wright, a primatologist with New York State's Stony Brook University commented that "It's exciting to watch these chimps do something that we've seen only people do before—use their feet to push the stick into the ground as a farmer might do with a shovel."

Even lower primates have shown higher mentality than expected in recently devised tests. Last year, capuchin monkeys were taught to swap tokens for food.

Fair Is Fair

"Normally, capuchins were happy to exchange their tokens for cucumber. But if one monkey was given a cucumber while the other got a (tastier) grape for the same token, the first monkey rebelled. Some refused to pay, others took the cucumber but refused to eat it. The animal's umbrage was even greater if the other monkey was rewarded for doing nothing. They did more than sulk, sometimes throwing the food out of their cage," reported the *Telegraph.* "The capuchin study reveals an emotional sense of fairness plays a key role in [economic] decision-making," said Sarah Brosnan of the Yerkes National Primate Research Centre of Emory University. This sense of equality may be common among social primates, the article added.

And while it's often easy to see, and easy for human supremacists to concede, similarities between our behavior and that of other primates, people who ascribe what are considered human characteristics to their animal companions are known to be, and cautioned for, "anthropomorphizing."

Or at least they were—one of the key assertions that cat and dog people make, that their animals have distinct personalities, has just been scientifically established.

Now It's Person-Al

Discovery News reported late last year about a cross-species personality published in the *Journal of Personality and Social Psychology,* showing that dogs have personalities, and that these character traits can be identified as accurately as similar personality attributes in humans. "Dogs," the article notes, "were chosen because of their wide availability, the fact that they safely and naturally exhibit a wide variety of behaviors, are understood well by many humans, and can travel to research sites with ease. Experts, however, suspect that many other animals also possess unique personalities."

Well, personalities, yes, but can dogs think? Now, whether the dog who recently saved her owner's life by calling 911 and barking incessantly into the phone receiver was "thinking" may be arguable.

Certainly the puppy who managed to shoot the man who was killing the whole litter was just a lucky shot. But these anecdotes, and others, are not the only indications of the capabilities of companion animals.

In June, the journal *Science* reported that "A German border collie named Rico has learned 200 words, indicating that a dog's ability to understand language is far better than expected." A *Bloomberg News* story goes on to explain that Rico "correctly retrieved 37 out of 40 toys by name." Here's the kicker: "The dog was given the names of the toys just once."

OK: Do you speak German? If so, pick another language, but if not . . . let's pretend you're given German words for 40 objects, hearing each word only once. Would you then be able to match more than 37 of them?

I'm pretty sure most non-German speakers, including me, wouldn't even come close. What does that tell us?

Any one of these incidents puts a serious dent in the concept of human supremacy, if only because it shows that our previous assumption about the line delineating human consciousness from (nonhuman) animal consciousness is not where we thought it was, and calls into question our ability to judge the issue dispassionately. But the pull of speciesism is strong, and the human brain is powerful and adaptable enough to generate new rationalizations on the fly: Primates are close to us genetically, and dogs and cats are close to us domestically, so sure, those animals might be the exceptions that prove the rule, but the rule still stands: You don't see other, "lower" animals making tools, for instance.

Bird Brains

But even that assurance was torpedoed earlier this century, when "Betty the Crow" surprised tool-usage researchers by making her own tool to complete a task. Researchers wondered whether she would know to pick a hooked wire rather than a straight one to successfully lift a small jar from a tube to get at food. When her companion flew off with the hooked wire, Betty took the straight wire and bent it into a hook and retrieved the food—then she repeated this nine out of ten times in subsequent experiments.

In short, all this time it may have been our own inability to measure and comprehend the thought processes of birds (for instance) that has made the expression "bird brain" so derogatory. A recent *Christian Science Monitor* article begins with a humorous admission of this: "Bird brains seem to be smarter these days." Less ironically, it continues: "Scientists are finding hints of a higher level of intelligence than expected as they look more closely at our avian friends." A pair of studies on finches and jays showed the birds grasping more about their social situation and acting more upon it than scientists had assumed they could.

Doors of Perception?

Similarly, news from the world of squirrels shows that there may be realms of intellect, socializing, and language that we have so far not been privy to because they work, literally, on a different wavelength. Using video cameras and a special ultrasonic device, Canadian researchers discovered that Richardson's ground squirrels were warning each other about predators by means of high-pitched squeals inaudible to humans and probably to most of the squirrels' predators as well. "They're able to discriminate among callers based on their calls, and they can communicate fairly specific information," said zoologist David Wilson, who speculates that the content of the squirrels' vocalizing "may include detailed information about the squirrels' predators."

A similarly-constructed study reported in November found sea animals virtually translating what entirely different species are saying: Seals, dolphins, and other marine mammals listen to the voice patterns of killer whales and can distinguish between two social classes of the same species of whale, knowing when to get out of the way of those that are hunting. An article in *Discovery* says these findings "could suggest marine mammals translate what the whales are saying," and although lead author Volker Deecke resists putting it that strongly, he does allow that "forest monkeys can decipher the alarm call of another monkey species, and hornbills, a tropical forest bird, can decipher monkey and eagle alarm calls." The question might arise of how well human efforts to decipher other animals' communication compare with these.

One line of delineation that persists even in discussion by some animal rights activists essentially excludes farm animals from true consideration in the intellectual community. Unsurprisingly, not many cognitive experiments are done on Holsteins or pigs. But even our poster child for the concept of "dumb animal," the sheep, has been shown to be able to remember up to 50 different sheep faces for more than two years, as well as recognizing human faces. (And how many sheep faces can you tell apart, by the way?)

And the more we look at even "lower" animals than that, the more we discover about the limitations of our own understanding. Fish, it turns out, "possess cognitive abilities outstripping those of some small mammals," reports the *Sunday Telegraph*. With tests of memory and cognition that had previously been untried, Dr. Theresa Burt de Perera found that fish are "very capable of learning and remembering, and possess a range of cognitive skills that would surprise many people."

Self-Conscious

Well, no matter what, we can fall back on our unique sense of self, though, right? Animals may be conscious of many things in the world around them, more things than we may have previously recognized, but we're still unique because we are aware of our own consciousness—we can think about thinking, a "cognitive self-awareness" that is unknown in other animals.

Or rather, was unknown, until we made a real effort to look for it.

"The Comparative Psychology of Uncertainty Monitoring and Metacognition," in the *Journal of Behavior and Brain Sciences,* describes three studies with humans, a group of Rhesus monkeys and one bottlenose dolphin using memory trials. Any animal that didn't want to complete a particular trial could respond "uncertain." It turned out that the monkeys and the dolphin used the "uncertain" response in a pattern "essentially identical to the pattern with which uncertain humans use it." Indeed, head researcher David Smith said that "the patterns of results produced by humans and animals provide some of the closest human-animal similarities in performance ever reported in the comparative literature." He added that the results "suggest that some animals have functional features of, or parallels to, human conscious metacognition."

In other words, science has repeatedly shown us that our basis for classifying our species as unique and supreme is more thoroughly based in human chauvinism than in factual reality. Ironically, we seem to be irrational about defending our rationality. But why would this be?

Of course part of the problem is the way these "surprising" studies are conveyed, with each scientist proudly (jealously?) proclaiming a conventional-wisdom-busting breakthrough as though no others had occurred, and the mainstream media delivering the story to us as "quirky" or "odd" devoid of larger context.

But the other part is that most humans don't want to entertain the possibility that other animals share most of the characteristics we think of as uniquely human. That's because it's only by thinking of animals as unthinking, unfeeling automatons—by insisting that the sun still revolves around the earth—that we can shrug off the enormous harm that our species perpetrates on other animals, cruelly and unnecessarily, each and every day.

If we are to make a case for ourselves as uniquely conscious, the most logical way to prove that might be to abandon "human supremacy" and behave in a way that shows we grasp the larger implications of our species' actions: To restore ecosystems instead of destroying them; to eat what's best in the long run for our bodies and our ideals, instead of what's most immediately handy; to instill in our children a respect for all forms of sentient life.

It's possible, of course, that we could subsequently find that some animal somewhere has, in some way, done the same thing, once again redrawing the line.

But the effort would not be wasted: At the very least we would have finally lived up to and embodied the term we use to describe ourselves:

Humanity.

References

Chimps Shown Using Not Just a Tool but a "Tool Kit," *National Geographic News,* 10/6/04

Capuchins Prove We Are Brothers under the Skin, *The Telegraph (UK),* 9/18/03

Study: Dogs Have Personalities, *Discovery News,* 12/11/03

Four-Legged Lifesaver, *Tri-City Herald,* 10/29/04

Pup Shoots Man, Saves Litter Mates, *Associated Press,* 9/9/04

Dogs Understand Language Better than Expected, Study Finds, *Bloomberg News,* 6/10/04

Crow Makes Wire Hook to Get Food, *National Geographic News,* 8/8/02

Intelligence? It's for the Birds, *Christian Science Monitor,* 9/2/04

Ground Squirrels Scream Ultrasonic Warning, *CBC News,* 7/29/04

Marine Mammals Eavesdrop on Orcas, *Discovery News,* 11/12/04

Study Shows Sheep Have Keen Memory for Faces, *Scientific American*, 11/9/01

Fast-Learning Fish Have Memories That Put Their Owners to Shame, *The Telegraph (UK)*, 10/3/04

New UB Research Finds Some Animals Know Their Cognitive Limits, *University at Buffalo Reporter*, 12/11/03

Appendix
"Leftovers" Lyrics

Whaddaya live on? Whaddaya do without meat? Whaddaya got left to eat?

Well, there's
Broccoli Gingerbread Almonds and Rice Milk for your Corn Flakes
Asparagus Artichokes Apricot Agar Pineapple and Carrot Cake
Banana Biscotti Sorbet Manicotti and Raisins and Strawberry Waffles
Tomatoes Potatoes Gazpacho and Nachos Alfalfa Fennel and Falafel
There's
Coconut Baklava Cucumber Sesame Chili and Chutney and Cherries
And Chickpeas Cilantro Polenta Pimento Pistachio Pesto and Blueberries
There's
Peaches and Apples and Nectarines—Cornbread and Cabbage and Collard Greens
Lentils and Pintos and Navy Beans—Lemons and Tangerines

With so many treats so neat complete and sweet to eat why bother to have a cow?

There's
Cinnamon Grapes Avocadoes and Dates Peanut Butter and Raspberry Jam
A Roll Guacamole Granola Stromboli Tabouli and Cole Slaw and Yams

Mangoes Tamales Oatmeal Macadamias Marzipan Tea Cauliflower
And Mint Macaroni Miso Minestrone French Onion and Soup Hot & Sour
There's
Kiwi and Ziti and Seaweed Fajitas and Pizzas and Beets and Raita
And Leeks Fettuccini Sushimi Rotini and Baba Ganoush on a Pita
There's
Pralines and Pretzels and Plantain Chips—Pickles and Pea Soup and Licorice Whips
Garlic and Mushroom Asparagus Tips—Cumin and Black Bean Dip

With so many treats so neat complete and sweet to eat why bother to have a cow?
With so many treats so neat complete and sweet to eat why bother another cow?

There's
Hummus Okra Tacos Salsa Spinach Curry Bagels Enchiladas Ratatouille Ketchup
Lettuce Seitan Olives Pasta Salad Tempeh Stuffin'
Veggie Burgers Watermelon Portabellos Bean Burritos Bulgur Pilaf Quesadillas
Apple Cider Orange Turnips and Cranberry Muffin
Walnuts Currants Orzo Radishes and Rhubarb Grits Spaghetti Biscuit Cantaloupe Risotto
Lemonade Balsamic Vinaigrette Papaya Hoagies
And Couscous Vermicelli Jalapenos Nutmeg Kale Lasagna Mustard Popcorn Sweet Potato
Pears Pecan Party Mix Plum Pottage Pumpkin Pierogies

A Veggie Pot Pie or a Barley Stew—Tempura Stir-Fry Marinated Tofu
Buckwheat and Brussels Sprouts Borscht Bok Choy

(And don't forget *The Joy of Soy*)
Green Tortellini Gnocchi Zucchini Rotelle Tahini Tostadas Linguini

With so many treats so neat complete and sweet to eat why bother to have a cow?
That's what we live on, that's what we do without meat,
That's what there is left to eat
It's called food.

CPSIA information can be obtained
at www.ICGtesting.com
Printed in the USA
FFOW02n1150230616
25296FF